"No pulse, no breathing," she whispered. She pressed the send key on her radio. "45–12 to all units. Code 99." A confirmed cardiac arrest. "The patient's a boy aged about seven. Expedite."

"He's only six," Mrs. Donaldson whispered.

Pam got onto her knees and found her hand position for chest compressions on the boy's small chest. "One, two, three, four, five." She gave a breath. "One, two, three, four, five." She gave another breath. Slowly she switched into autopilot, compressing, then giving breaths. After about a minute, she leaned over and again checked the boy's pulse and breathing. Surprised, she thought she felt a faint pulse. She checked again. The pulse was weak, but it was definitely there. "Thank you, God," she whispered. But the boy still wasn't breathing. . . .

By Joan E. Lloyd and Edwin B. Herman:

RESCUE ALERT
DIAL 911*
LIGHTS AND SIREN*
TRAUMA CENTER*

*Published by Ivy Books

Books published by The Ballantine Publishing Group
are available at quantity discounts on bulk purchases
for premium, educational, fund-raising, and special
sales use. For details, please call 1-800-733-3000.

TRAUMA CENTER

**Joan E. Lloyd
and
Edwin B. Herman**

IVY BOOKS • NEW YORK

An Ivy Book
Published by Ballantine Books
Copyright © 1997 by Joan E. Lloyd and Edwin B. Herman

All rights reserved under International and Pan-American Copyright Conventions. Published in the United States by Ballantine
Books, a division of Random House, Inc., New York, and simultaneously in Canada by Random House of Canada Limited, Toronto.

http://www.randomhouse.com

Library of Congress Catalog Card Number: 97-93781

ISBN 0-8041-1546-X

Manufactured in the United States of America

First Edition: November 1997

10 9 8 7 6 5 4 3 2

To the members of the Yorktown Volunteer Ambulance Corps and the Mohegan Volunteer Fire Association, with whom we have shared well over a thousand good, bad, and strange calls over the years:

Thank you for your help, support, and camaraderie. We have laughed with you, cried with you, and have benefited greatly from your professionalism, your caring, and your dedication.

Acknowledgments

We would like to acknowledge the help of the following organizations:

Hudson Valley Hospital Center, Peekskill, New York
Key West Rescue, Key West, Florida
Med Star Ambulance Services, Savannah, Georgia
The Northern Westchester Hospital Center, Mount Kisco, New York
Palm Beach County Search and Rescue, Palm Beach, Florida
Stat Flight, Valhalla, New York
The Westchester County Medical Center, Valhalla, New York

We would also like to thank our editor Elisa Wares and our agent Meg Ruley for their continuing help, support, and encouragement.

Chapter 1

Seventeen-year-old Josh Evans was still angry with his best friend, Cory. "Sandy got the day off and we're going to the movies," Cory had told him on the phone the previous evening.

"But what about our hike?"

"Oh, come on, Josh. You understand. When Sandy gets the day off, I want to be with her."

"Cory's such a shit. Girls," Josh muttered at the breakfast table the following morning. Of course, if he had the opportunity to go somewhere with Amanda McCarthy . . .

"What's the matter, Josh?" his mother asked, then forked some pancakes into her mouth.

"Nothing. It's just that Cory isn't going with me today. He's got other plans." His lip curled. "He finked out at the last minute."

"That's too bad. What will you do today instead?"

"I'm going to climb anyway. I've had it planned for weeks."

"You're not climbing Miller's Crag alone, and that's final," Josh's father said, around a mouthful of bacon.

"Oh, come on, Dad, be real. I've climbed it before."

1

"I don't care, you're not going alone. It's too dangerous."

"It's not a bad climb," Josh said, now not caring as much about the climb as about the point to be made. No one was going to tell him what to do and what not to do. Particularly his parents.

"Brad," Mrs. Evans said to Josh's father, "maybe we can compromise."

"It's too dangerous. He's not going all alone, and that's final."

Mrs. Evans turned to Josh. "What if there's trouble? After all, what if you get bitten by a snake and there's no one around?"

"Oh, Mom. There are no poisonous snakes on Miller's Crag."

"Your father and I would worry. But maybe if you take my cell phone . . ."

Josh wanted to carry the cell phone like he wanted a third foot.

"That's not good enough," his father said firmly.

"Now, come on, dear," Mrs. Evans said to her husband. "That way he can call if he gets into any difficulties."

Josh kept his face angled down into his plate and listened to his parents argue about him as if he weren't there. He had long ago figured out his parents' dynamics, so Josh sat quietly and let his mother fight his battle for him. That was how he had gotten his driver's license and had been able to buy his car, a seven-year-old Plymouth.

"That cell phone of yours doesn't make a difference," his father said, getting that no-one's-going-to-tell-me-what-my-son-can-do tone in his voice. "He isn't going."

Josh could see that his mother was backing down this time, so he stepped in. "Come on, Dad. You and I have climbed Miller's Crag together and I know the area real well. I'm not a kid anymore. Stop treating me like a baby. I've got my own car and I'll be a senior next year."

Mr. Evans looked up and stared at his son for a long time. "All right, Josh," his father said with a sigh. "You're right."

Holy shit! Josh thought. Will wonders never cease?

"But you take that cell phone."

Knowing that he wouldn't get out of the dining room without the damn phone, Josh said, "Thanks, Dad, Mom." He stuffed the last mouthful of his mom's pancakes into his mouth.

"Shall I pack you a sandwich?" she asked.

"Sure. Thanks, Mom. And throw in a bag of chips and a few Cokes too."

Half an hour later, his mother handed him his back-pack, stuffed with food, sodas, and the cell phone. "You know how to use that phone," she said. "But no personal calls. Those cost a fortune."

Because it was expected, Josh kissed his mother on the cheek, then headed off.

Miller's Crag was a seventeen-hundred-foot-high peak about an hour's drive from Josh's house. The lower part was forested, criss-crossed by trails and easy to climb. Above there was a steep but hikeable trail over the bare, rocky slope. In a few places it was necessary to climb over rubble from a small rockslide that had occurred the previous summer. The trail ended at a flattened area at the summit where hikers picnicked and enjoyed a superb view of most of the county.

When Josh arrived at the foot of the crag, he considered not bothering with the climb at all. Why should I do this? he mused. I could just drive around and see which of the guys want to hang out. Without Cory it isn't really going to be any fun anyway. Then he spotted a group of high school girls in hiking boots with backpacks and water bottles climbing out of a van at the far end of the parking area. "Oh, what the hell. I'm here anyway."

About halfway up the lower section he passed the five girls. "Hi there," he said.

A few of the girls said hi as he tramped past them. "See ya at the top," Josh called back to them. Then, to demonstrate what good shape he was in, Josh took off rapidly up the slope.

At about eleven hundred feet, the trail got steeper and rockier. Josh paused for a few minutes, drank a soda, and stuffed the empty can into his backpack. Then he decided to move off the trail and take a slightly different line up the rock-strewn slope. While climbing, however, he realized that his new course took him up some particularly steep areas. As he reached for a handhold, one foot slipped on some loose rubble; flailing his arms and legs, he slipped, bounced, and slithered down the slope and off the edge of a steep embankment.

When the world came back into focus, Josh realized that he was lying on his left side, pressed against the small tree that must have stopped his descent, pillowed half on, half off his backpack. He looked up and saw that he was about two-thirds of the way down the steep slope, about fifty feet below the ledge from which he had fallen. He lay in a wooded area, surrounded by small trees and thick scrub. "Shit, shit, shit," he muttered, then took slow, shallow breaths trying to calm his pounding heart. I'm okay, he told himself. I'm okay. I just need a minute to catch my breath. Covered with scratches and feeling very bruised, he slowly tried to sit up, but an excruciating pain stabbed through his hips and down his left leg. He collapsed back into the position he had found himself in moments earlier, his shirt shredded and blood flowing from several deep lacerations.

"Okay, man," he said aloud. "Let me check this out." He felt along his right leg as he had seen the doctors do in medical programs he enjoyed on TV. There was no pain there, but when he reached for his left leg, the pain almost made him throw up. "Broke my fuckin' leg. Shit, shit, shit." As he lay back down and tried to calm his breathing and his stomach, the seriousness of his situa- tion began to seep into his mind. Since the sound of his own voice was comforting, he spoke aloud. "No one can see me. I'm too buried in these trees. I can't move to get help. I'm such a fuckin' jerk."

Then he remembered the phone.

It took almost five minutes of tiny movements to maneuver the backpack from beneath him. "Don't be smashed, you shit," he mumbled as he rummaged in the pack. On quick inspection the phone seemed to be fine. He pulled up the antenna and pressed the POWER button. The screen appeared and the words "No service" flashed while the instrument searched for a transmitter. "Come on, find something," Josh said.

Three lines appeared on the screen. "Yes," Josh hissed, knowing that he could indeed make a call. He dialed 911.

"911," a woman's voice said.

"I need help," Josh said; then, to his chagrin, he started to cry.

"Okay, we can help." The woman's voice sounded supportive and kind. "What's the problem?"

Josh swallowed hard. "I fell and I'm hurt real bad. It's my leg, and I'm bleeding all over."

"Okay, tell me your name."

"Josh." His voice sounded small and scared.

"Josh what?"

"Evans. Josh Evans."

"Good, Josh. My name's Pam. How old are you, Josh?"

"I'm seventeen."

"Where are you?"

"I was climbing Miller's Crag and . . ." He swallowed hard and tried not to let tears overwhelm him. ". . . and I went off to the left of the main trail. My foot slipped and I slid and rolled most of the way down. It hurts real bad."

"Josh, hold a moment while I get the state police and an ambulance on the way. I'll be right back; don't hang up."

As the phone became silent, Josh felt very much alone. "Come back, lady," he said, tears rolling down his cheeks. He swiped them away with his tattered sleeve. "Come back, Pam, please."

"Okay, Josh," the voice said, "I'm back now. The police and an ambulance are on the way to you. Give me your cell phone number so we can stay in touch with you."

Josh remembered that his mother had programmed her own number into the machine under the code number 23 for her birthday. "It might make some noise, lady, but the number's in the phone." He pressed the buttons and read the number off to the 911 dispatcher.

"Good, Josh. Now, will they have trouble seeing you from the trail?"

Josh looked up. Leaves and branches. "They'll never

see me. I'm in the woods about two-thirds of the way down the slope."

"They will find you. They're trained to get people like you out of difficult places. They *will* find you."

"I hope so."

"Listen, Josh," Pam said. "You'd better hang up now. I usually keep people on the line, but I'm afraid of using up the batteries in your phone. We'll need to talk to you later when the ambulance is closer. I hate to leave you, but it's really best."

"I understand," Josh said, rubbing at the tears still rolling down his cheeks. "Good-bye." He pressed the END button on the phone and listened to the resulting silence. Then he placed the phone on the leaf-littered ground beside him, pillowed his head on his aching arm, and tried not to panic. Between the throb in his leg and hip and the pains and aches from his cuts and bruises, every minute passed like an hour.

Carrie VanWyk looked out through the plastic windows of the helicopter as it lifted from the pad behind the trauma center. "Air One to county control," Jeff Marks, the pilot, said into the mike. "We are code 100."

Sharon Blackstone, the second flight nurse on duty that day, sat beside Carrie. "Poor kid," she said. "Control says he's hurt pretty bad."

"I've been on scene calls in that area before," Carrie said. "At least one person falls down that embankment each year." She looked at her partner. "But at least this one had a cell phone."

"Yeah, I heard. That's amazing. So many of these idiots go off alone and have no way to get help if they get in trouble."

Since it was impossible to hear inside the helicopter, all communications among members of the crew came through their radio. Jeff's voice came through Carrie's earphones. "Get me the frequency of the local ground control, will you, Carrie?"

"Sure." She keyed the mike on the panel on the wall at her side. "County from Air One."

"County."

"Can you give us info about ground command at the scene?"

"Command will be Chief Burke of the Miller Pond Fire Department." Then he gave the appropriate radio frequency. "What's your ETA?"

"ETA about twenty minutes."

"10–4 Air One. Let me know when you're on the ground."

"10–4." Carrie replaced the mike in the holder and adjusted her heavy helmet. "Poor kid," she said softly.

Nineteen minutes later Air One was over the collection of fire trucks and volunteer vehicles that crowded the parking area at the foot of Miller's Crag.

"Ground to Air One."

"Go ahead, ground," Jeff said.

"We need your help from the air. I'm Chief Burke of the Miller Pond Fire Department. I need you to locate my vehicle. I'll turn on my blue light."

Carrie saw a light flash on. "There." She pointed and saw Jeff nod.

"Got it."

"Good. The kid's in a heavily wooded section that starts about half a mile due north of my car. We need a more precise location. Since I have his cell phone number, I'll call him and have him tell us when you're directly overhead. Just fly over slowly, and I'll tell you when he tells me. Then you can give us a fix."

"Will do," Jeff said, and headed due north.

Josh glanced at his watch again. It had been almost twenty-five minutes since he had hung up the phone and now he wasn't feeling so well. He was sweaty, weak, and a bit nauseous. As he took a deep breath to try to clear his head, he heard two sounds almost simultaneously. First was the unmistakable whirring of a helicopter; second was the ringing of his phone. He pushed the SEND button and heard a man's voice. "Josh?"

"Yeah." He tried not to sound as wimpy as he felt but didn't think he was doing a particularly good job. "I'm here."

"I'm Chief Burke. Most of my friends just call me Chief. We're going to get you out of there."

"I'm really glad to hear from you, Chief."

"I'm glad to hear you too. How are you feeling?"

"I'm okay," he said, hoping he would believe it.

"Josh, we've got a helicopter overhead. Can you hear it?"

"Yeah."

"Here's what we want you to do. They'll fly above you very slowly. Can you see the sky straight up?"

Slowly Josh turned his head so he could look up out of the corner of his eye. "Yeah."

"Watch and tell me when you see the chopper right overhead. Then we'll know just where you are."

"Okay." Josh waited and listened to the helicopter. "It sounds like it's going away from me now," he said a minute later.

"Good boy. I'll tell them." Josh heard the chief tell the

helicopter to turn around. If I wasn't in so much pain, Josh thought, this would be really neat.

As the sound got louder again, Josh stared up through a small opening in the leaves. Then he saw it. "Yeah. I see it. It's right above me." Through the phone he heard a small cheer.

"Josh," the chief said, "you're about a mile from here and up about two hundred feet. We're going to get some equipment together, and we'll probably be there in about half an hour. I know that seems like a long time but you can be sure we're going as fast as we can. Okay?"

Half an hour. It seemed like forever, but there was nothing he could do to make it happen any sooner. "Okay," Josh said.

"Good boy."

"Did anyone call my folks?"

"They're on their way right now. They should be here about the same time we get to you."

Quietly Josh said, "They'll kill me."

"No, they won't, Josh. They'll be so glad you're okay that they'll forget to be mad."

Despite his pains, Josh grinned. "You don't know my folks."

"Don't worry. I'll see to it that they're nice to you or they'll answer to me."

"Thanks."

"Save your battery and hang up now. We'll be there real soon."

Reluctantly Josh pushed the END button.

On the ground to one side of the parking lot, Carrie, Sharon, and Jeff had little to do but wait. Another helicopter that was in service would respond to any other

serious accident calls. From now on they were committed to Josh. Although they could do more than the
local ambulance crew, Carrie assumed that the ambulance personnel would care for Josh and bring him to
the chopper for transport. While the pilot showed two
firefighters around the chopper, the two flight nurses
sat on the step of the fire rescue truck and chatted
with other volunteers. They watched the rescuers gather
ropes, a Stokes basket, a trauma kit, and immobilization
equipment.

A young woman from the ambulance crew walked
over. "One of you want to go with us? We could sure use
your help. The kid doesn't sound too good."

Carrie looked at Sharon. "I'll go," they said in unison.
"You stay here," Carrie said. "I'm in the mood for a
walk." She went back to the chopper and got the IV bag
and the airway roll. Within moments, Carrie and seven
turnout-coated rescuers headed out across the parking lot
in the direction of Josh's position.

Fifteen minutes later Josh's phone rang. "Hello?"

"It's Chief Burke again, Josh. How are you doing?"

"I'm okay," he said, feeling really rotten. It was taking
a great effort now not to throw up.

"We're trying to zero in on you. Can you see the slope
from where you are? Do you know uphill from down?"

"Yeah."

"I'm going to yell real loud. Let me know whether
you can hear me."

Through the trees Josh heard a distant voice calling
"Hello."

"I hear you," he said into the phone.

"Great. Which way is my voice? Are we downhill
from you?"

"Yeah." Josh tried to gather his thoughts. They were too far to the east. "If you're looking uphill, you need to move more to your left, to the west."

"Good boy. We're coming toward you right now. Do you know how to check the battery power in the phone?"

"I think so." Josh pushed the FUNCTION button, then entered the code for battery power. "It's okay. The battery's okay."

"Good, then stay on the line with me."

Twice more the chief yelled and Josh gave him directions. Suddenly Josh heard the sounds of men crashing through the trees. "I hear you. You're right here." He put the phone aside and yelled, "Here I am!"

"We got you," the chief yelled. Several men in black-and-yellow fire department coats appeared. A big, beefy man crouched at Josh's side. "Hi, Josh, I'm Chief Burke."

Trying not to sob, Josh said, "I'm real glad to see you."

A woman in a bright red jumpsuit appeared beside the chief, who quickly moved aside. "Hi, Josh. I'm Carrie and I'm a flight nurse. That was my helicopter you heard." While she talked she took Josh's wrist as one of the men held his head.

Despite his pain and nausea, he was fascinated by the idea of riding in a helicopter. "Wow. I've never been in a helicopter." Josh watched as Carrie took her stethoscope, pressed the end against his chest, and made him breathe several times.

"You might just get to ride with us. But for now, you just rest and let us take good care of you. Wiggle your fingers for me, can you?" He did. "And your toes?"

"It hurts when I move my left foot." Josh wiggled the toes on his right foot.

Carrie reached over and squeezed his sneaker. "Which toe am I touching?"

"The big one."

"That's real good."

"Boy, I'm glad you're here."

"Squeeze my hands," Carrie said, and Josh took her hands and squeezed.

"Good boy." Without moving Josh from his side, Carrie began a thorough, head-to-toe exam. "I'm checking to see what's broken," she told him.

"It's my leg."

"Which one?" Carrie asked, checking his head and neck for injuries.

"My left. Hurts real bad when I move."

"Then don't move. That's an important rule." As she spoke she palpated his ribs. "Take a deep breath for me." When he did, she asked, "Did it hurt when you did that?"

"No. What's an important rule?"

As Carrie palpated Josh's abdomen, she said, "An important rule of emergency medicine. But it's very secret. Do you still want to hear it?"

Josh's eyes widened. "Sure." He watched all the medical shows on TV and wanted to know all the good stuff.

"You tell me if anything I do hurts and I'll tell you all my secrets." She placed one hand on each of Josh's hip bones and pressed gently but firmly.

Josh gasped. "That hurts a lot."

"I gather." Good chance of a pelvic fracture, she thought, and filed the information away for later. "I won't do it again. Well, the first rule is 'If it hurts when you do that, don't do it.' " She worked her way down his right leg, hoping there was no pain there. There wasn't.

Very seriously, Josh said, "That makes sense."

"Yeah, it does. That leg seems okay."

Not wanting to embarrass the flight nurse, Josh said softly, "I said it was the other one."

Carrie grinned. "I know. I always check the good one first."

"Why?"

"Because if I check the bad one first, it might hurt so much you wouldn't know whether the good one hurt too."

"Oh."

"I'm going to check the bad one now. It might hurt."

"I'm ready."

Carrie ran her trained hands down Josh's injured leg. "Ow," he yelled as her hands pressed below his knee.

"I think this is broken," she said, not hiding information from her patient. She took her shears and split Josh's left jeans leg from ankle to hip. Even though the boy was lying on his side, Carrie could see that there was obvious deformity in the middle of his lower leg. "We call this the tib-fib," she told him. One of the EMTs handed her a foldable splint but she shook her head. They could splint Josh only when he was turned on his back. It would be best to do all the movement at once. "There are two bones in the lower leg. One is called the fibula and one called the tibia. Since we don't know which is broken until we get X rays, we just say tib-fib."

"Tib-fib. That's like a broken leg."

"That's a broken leg," Carrie said. A backboard lay on the ground beside the boy and two firefighters brought up the Stokes, a heavy wire-mesh basket large enough for Josh's entire body, on the backboard, to be cradled and carried. Carrie knew that once they had him on the board, splinted, and in the basket, he would be more protected and a bit more comfortable.

On her nod, one of the ambulance crew members fastened a collar around Josh's neck. "That's to protect you. I know it's not too comfortable, but we really need to do it."

"I've seen this on *Rescue 911*," Josh said. "They always do this to people who fall or are in car crashes."

"Ah, so you watch *Rescue 911*. Well, you'll have to check us out and see that we're doing all this right." Carrie rechecked his pulse and decided not to start an IV line until later. "Josh," she said, "we are going to have to move you, and I'll tell you right now it won't be comfortable. We'll try to be as gentle as we can so just hold on."

"Okay."

"Don't help. Let us do all the work." She looked at the panic in the boy's eyes and took his hand. "When we move you, you just squeeze as hard as you can." She looked at the three men who had positioned themselves behind Josh. They took the six-foot-long backboard and laid it on the ground against the boy's back. "We're going to roll you from your side onto the board behind you." She first looked at the EMT near Josh's knees. On the long walk up the hill she had learned his name. "Kent," she said, "can you support Josh's leg? Be really careful, because this is going to hurt like crazy."

"Got it," Kent said.

Then she looked at the firefighter holding Josh's head. "I'm sorry," she said, "I don't know your name."

"I'm Bob," the man said.

"Okay, Bob, on your count."

"One, two, three." While Bob held Josh's head and

Kent supported his injured leg, three other firefighters rolled the boy from his left side onto the long backboard.

As his body moved, Josh couldn't suppress the scream. As he cried out, Carrie felt his death grip on her hand as he squeezed as tightly as he could.

"The worst is over. Can you feel me touching your foot?" she asked, pinching his left big toe again.

"Yeah."

She quickly found his pedal pulse. "Good pulse and neurological function in this foot," she told him. She slipped the foldable splint onto Josh's leg, until it covered him from midthigh to toes, then used the Velcro straps to fasten it tightly. Again she checked his foot and found everything unchanged. "All right," she said.

As the men fastened several straps tightly over Josh's body and taped head-immobilizing plastic blocks against the sides of his head, Carrie watched Josh's face relax. "Better?" she said softly.

"That hurt."

Carrie reached into her pocket and handed Josh a tissue. "No one's watching," she whispered. With a small smile, Josh wiped the tears from his face. "Okay, babe," Carrie said. "I'm going to start an IV line just like you see them do on TV." It took only moments to get the line started and check Josh's vitals. "Now let's put these guys to work carrying you out of here."

The firefighters had rigged long ropes for handholds along the trail they had blazed on the way up, and within twenty minutes the group was back on level ground. As they walked toward the waiting helicopter, two people, obviously Josh's parents, arrived. "Josh, baby," his mother cried, looking into the Stokes basket. "Are you all right?"

"Sure, Mom, I'm fine," Josh said. Actually he *was* feeling a bit better. At least the nausea had subsided.

"We were petrified." The woman turned to Carrie. "Is he really all right?"

"Tell them about your leg, Josh," Carrie said.

"I've got a broken tib-fib."

"Oh, my God," Josh's mother said. "What's that?"

"Oh, Mom," Josh said, "it's just my leg. I broke my leg."

"Anything else?"

"On the way down the mountain, Carrie told me I might have a pelvic fracture. That's right here." Josh slipped one arm out of the strap that held him fast to the long backboard and pointed to his hip. "Right there."

"But you're all covered with blood." His mother's eyes were wide and her breathing was rapid.

Carrie stepped in. "He's taken a bad fall and he's got lots of cuts and bruises. From what I can tell, however, I think his leg and pelvis are the worst of his injuries. The rest is superficial."

"Are you sure?" his mother asked.

"We'll take him to the hospital and they'll examine him and take X rays. You know, he's quite a boy, Mrs. Evans. He called 911 on his cell phone and helped us find him."

"He did?"

"He certainly did," Carrie said, patting Mrs. Evans on the hand. "He's a great kid."

Mr. Evans spoke for the first time. "See? Best idea I ever had. I'm glad I insisted that you bring that phone."

"*You* insisted?" Mrs Evans said. "Hogwash. It was my idea."

As the two argued, Carrie and Pete loaded Josh into the helicopter. "Josh is going to St. Luke's Trauma Center in Oakmont. You two will have to drive there, but we're going for a helicopter ride."

"Awesome," Josh said, as Carrie climbed in behind him.

"Can't I go with you?" Mrs. Evans said.

"No, I'm sorry. There's not enough room."

Josh beamed at the helicopter crew as his parents slowly walked back to their car. In the helicopter, Carrie put an oxygen mask over Josh's face, then put a pair of headphones over his ears. "Can you hear me now?" she asked.

"Yeah," Josh said.

"Well, it's going to get real noisy in here when Jeff starts the engine." At that moment Jeff started the twin turbines and soon the chopper lifted off. Carrie saw the disappointed look on Josh's face. "I'm sorry that you can't see too much from where you're lying, but I'll make a deal. Once you're better you can make a date with me and we can go for a ride in the chopper so you can see everything."

"Really?" Josh said, his eyes wide.

"Yes, really."

Exhausted, moments later Josh drifted off to sleep.

Josh underwent surgery to set his badly fractured leg but his pelvic fracture was not displaced so it was allowed to heal on its own. Three days later the boy was discharged into the care of his parents.

Welcome to the world of emergency response. Whether by helicopter, ambulance, fly car, or all-terrain vehicle, on horseback or on foot, every hour of every day, emergency medical technicians (EMTs), paramedics, and flight nurses speed to the scene of accidents and illnesses to render medical and psychological assistance. In emergency rooms all around the country, dedicated staff members continue care. Come into that world with us.

Throughout the pages of this book you will read about the experiences of real-life EMTs in the field and nurses and doctors in the emergency room. All the stories are based on actual events. In fact, most are derived from calls that Ed and I have responded to in our combined thirty-five years in emergency medical service (EMS). Some are based on situations drawn from the experiences of our friends and acquaintances, and a few are based on letters written by readers of our previous books. The hospital stories are culled from our years of relationships with emergency room personnel and from hours of volunteer service and observation.

Although all the tales in this book are based on fact, we have considered the privacy of our patients and associates. Therefore, Ed and I have fictionalized these stories sufficiently so that no one is recognizable. The towns in this book are fictional localities, based on the places in which we ride, as are the business establishments, stores, roadways, and the like. Fairfax Volunteer Ambulance Corps is a creation of our imagination, but the EMTs are modeled after our friends and associates. Fairfax General Hospital and St. Luke's Trauma Center are patterned after institutions in our area.

The fictional Fairfax Volunteer Ambulance Corps responds to over 1,500 calls a year. To staff three ambulances and answer that many calls for help, ordinarily an ambulance corps would need sixty or seventy EMT volunteers. In this book, however, we've used the same few people over and over again.

As you read, you'll learn about the equipment we use, the treatments we give, and the jargon we have adopted. If you're curious about any of these terms, check the glossary at the end of this book.

Most of the calls to which any EMT responds are routine, situations in which sick people are transported to the hospital. Because we want to describe the unusual and the dramatic, it may seem that we respond to an unusually high number of car accidents and other calls involving dramatic trauma. This isn't the real story of emergency medical work, just the more interesting part.

Emergency medical procedures change over time and vary from state to state, so we've used those of our particular area. At the time of this writing, all the procedures and protocols we describe are accurate. In addition, our stories and treatments frequently differ in several ways from those on popular TV shows.

First, we don't become good friends with our patients. Quite the contrary. Usually we see a slice of their lives, then never encounter them again.

Second, we don't stop doing CPR just so the camera can capture our expressions as we accept death. We cannot pronounce anyone dead. Rather, we continue caring for our patients in whatever way we can until we hand them off to the personnel in the helicopter or emergency room.

Third, we don't endanger our lives and the lives of those who might try to rescue us by putting ourselves into dangerous situations. We don't run into burning buildings, climb into unstable vehicles, or careen through red lights.

With those things in mind, turn the page and rejoin the real world of emergency medicine, in the field, in the ambulance, and in the trauma center.

Chapter 2

Charlie Woo, Mike Silverstein, and Joe Corelli had been friends for as long as any of them could remember. Neighbors, they had met in nursery school and had gone through Fairfax schools together, had tried out for sports together, and had gotten into their share of trouble together. Now, in mid-August after their senior year at Fairfax High School, the three friends were trying hard to get used to the idea of being separated. Charlie and Joe had been accepted at out-of-town schools while, due to his family's financial troubles, Mike had had to get a job and go to the local community college.

An unlikely trio, Charlie, Mike, and Joe were not only ethnically dissimilar but as physically different as three best friends could be. Charlie was small, scarcely five foot six, but with a well-developed upper body. Mike was tall and lanky, over six feet six inches. Joe was built like a barrel, five feet ten and more than 250 pounds.

It was a warm morning and the three young men had wrestled the top off Mike's Jeep and taken it out for a spin. Going nowhere in particular, they sped down the parkway toward the reservoir. "Hey," Charlie yelled to Mike from the passenger seat, "let's go north and head for Miller Pond." He motioned toward the bundle of clothes on the floor in the back. "We got towels and trunks."

"Yeah. Good idea." Joe leaned forward from the backseat and got his head between the headrests. "Let's stop at the deli and get sandwiches too."

"Always food," Mike yelled, slowing for the Route 42 exit. He turned off the parkway, whipped onto the northbound entrance ramp, and sped north toward Route 161. He took the appropriate exit ramp and, barely slowing for the full stop at the bottom, turned right toward town, across the path of a black Ford.

"Hey, man," Joe yelled as a horn blared, "you cut that bastard off pretty good."

"He had plenty of room. He just didn't want to touch his brake."

As they sped down Route 161, the Ford passed the Jeep and the driver flipped his middle finger out the open driver's side window as he pulled back into the lane and sped away.

"Fuckin' bastard," Mike yelled, stomping on the gas. As the speedometer passed fifty, Charlie braced his hands on the dashboard and Joe grabbed the roll bar. With both hands grasping the wheel, Mike pressed harder on the gas.

Suddenly, as the Jeep approached to within three car lengths, the Ford driver touched his brake and the distance between the two cars closed rapidly. "Shit," Mike screamed, and slammed his foot on the brake. Then the Ford accelerated, and the Jeep fishtailed. It crossed the road and the narrow verge and slammed into a tree, the point of impact slightly forward of the driver's side door.

When the car hit, Charlie was thrown from the passenger

seat. He flew about ten feet, and landed, facefirst, in a weed- and scrub-covered open area. Groggy and in a lot of pain, he lay still, trying to catch his breath, wondering whether he was going to live and hurting so badly that he was afraid he might.

Joe's well-padded body had slammed violently around the back of the Jeep. As he hung onto the roll bar with a death grip, he had watched Mike's body crash into the steering wheel then bounce against the side door. When the car came to rest, Joe found himself on the floor in the back of the Jeep. "Hey, Mike," Joe said as he struggled to sit up. He tried to catch his breath but he couldn't inhale without severe pain in his side. When Mike didn't answer, Joe tried to wiggle between the seats and get a look at his friend's face. What he saw was worse than anything he might have imagined. Mike was slumped against the driver's side door, his face covered with blood, his arm lying in his lap with the bone showing through a wide open gash.

Holding his side and unable to get his breath, Joe climbed out of the Jeep and staggered over to a car that had stopped at the scene. "Get help," he panted, unaware of the blood covering his forehead and cheeks. "Mike's real bad," he puffed, then, unable to stand any longer, he lay down on the grass at the side of the roadway.

Sandy Kowalski had been on her way to work as a receptionist at a printing firm when she saw the Jeep against the tree, wheels still spinning, spitting dirt onto the roadway. She pulled over, horrified at the sight of several injured teenagers. When one young man, covered with blood, ran up to the open passenger side window, she leaned toward him. "Get help," he yelled. Not knowing what else she could do, Sandy drove toward the Route 10 intersection where she knew there was a gas station and a phone booth.

Although I'm fifty-four and a gray-haired grand-mother, I am also a bit vain, so every week I have my nails done. It's an indulgence, but it's one I allow myself. It was ten twenty-five in the morning and Amy, one of the manicurists at Gala Nails, was just finishing the first coat of polish when the ambulance corps' tones went off. "Fairfax Police to the Ambulance Corps," we heard from my omnipresent two-way portable radio.

Hearing the ensuing silence, I could picture someone in the headquarters' kitchen getting up and walking to the microphone.

"You on duty today, Joan?" Amy asked.

"Nah. Not with wet nails. There's a full crew at head-quarters." Although not officially "on duty," I am basi-cally nosy and like to know what is going on. So I carry my Fairfax Volunteer Ambulance Corps portable radio clipped to the pocket of my jeans most of the time. In addition to my curiosity, I carry it because frequently I respond to calls when there is no duty crew available or when the duty crew is occupied on another call.

"Fairfax Ambulance on," said a voice I recognized as Linda Potemski's.

"The ambulance is needed at a PIAA at Route 161 and the parkway. Caller states there are serious injuries."

"10–4," Linda said. "45–01 is responding with a full crew. Let us know what the officer finds when he gets there."

Amy started the second coat of polish and said, "That's right near here. What's a PIAA?"

"That's a personal injury auto accident."

I was getting a bit impatient. I had already paid for my manicure and I was thinking of "jumping the call"—responding without being requested—a practice that's frowned on in Fairfax. So far, however, they hadn't called for a second rig. It might not be too serious.

"45–01 to Fairfax Police," Tom Franks's voice said. He must be driving. That probably meant that his wife, Heather, was on duty as well. Since both were part of the school system, they took advantage of the summer vacation to ride a few six-hour shifts a week, often together.

"Police on."

"Put the helicopter on standby."

"Helicopter," Amy said, finishing the second coat of polish on my right hand. "Does that mean it's really bad?"

"Not necessarily," I answered. "We put the chopper on standby when there's a report of serious injury. It just means that they will start the engines and assemble the crew. They won't fly unless the injuries warrant it."

"How do you handle all that blood and stuff?" Amy asked. Probably only in her early twenties, the blond manicurist always seemed to be wide-eyed about my work with the ambulance corps.

"I guess it's mostly that I've had a lot of practice, and I have hundreds of hours of training and routine to fall back on. When you know how to help, it's really easier than standing there with that helpless feeling I used to have before I got into emergency medical work."

As Amy finished the second coat of polish on my left hand, the radio sounded again. "Police to 45–01."

"45–01 on." We could hear the siren in the background.

"First officer on the scene asks that you expedite. There are at least three serious injuries."

"10–4. Tone out for another crew to respond to the scene with the second rig and get a third crew on standby. And alert Prescott."

"Prescott?" Amy asked.

"We have what's called a mutual aid system. If we don't have enough people, we can count on help from the neighboring districts. Prescott's closest, since one of their ambulances can get on the parkway southbound and be in our district in three minutes. They will get a standby crew ready in case we need them."

"But they said there are only three injuries," she said. "Why all this help?"

"The officer knows of three injuries, but it's amazing how many people think they're not injured until the excitement of the accident starts to wear off. Frequently they discover pains and aches five or ten minutes later. Or even hours later."

"Oh."

I watched Amy put the top on the polish and unscrew the lid on the bottle of top coat. "Frustrating," I muttered, "to have wet nails." I debated responding, wet nails and all, but decided to wait and see whether others were around to help. Often it's difficult to get people during weekdays, but in the summer many people are on vacation and might be eager to respond to a serious call like this.

"45–01 on location," Tom Franks's voice said.

"10–4, 45–01. Your time is ten fifty-three."

As Amy finished my right hand, I heard the rig radio. "45–01 to Fairfax Police. Have them launch the bird and get that second crew here stat."

"I'll tell control to launch the chopper," the dispatcher said. "I've only gotten a driver for the second rig so far."

"If you can't get a crew, have Prescott respond," Linda said. "We've got two serious and one critical."

I yanked my hand away from Amy and blowing on my nails, said, "Forget the rest. I'll be back later and you can redo whatever needs it." I grabbed my radio and sprinted toward my car. After keying my mike, I said, "45–24 to FPD."

"Go ahead, 24."

"I'm en route to the scene."

"10–4, Joan."

By the time I had put my green light on top of my car, started the engine, and driven from the parking lot, my nails were ruined. Mentally I shrugged. Oh, well. Just don't get that stuff on your T-shirt or your white jeans, I told myself.

Adrenaline is strong stuff. I could feel the powerful flight-or-fight hormone pound through my veins, insisting "Get there fast! Press on the gas!" My sane self overrode those commands. I know the risks run by anyone who speeds, especially through local residential streets. I've certainly seen enough of what poor driving can do in my twelve years in emergency medicine.

"45–22 to FPD." I recognized Ed's voice.

"Go ahead, unit calling."

"45–22 is en route. Do you need a driver at headquarters, or should I go to the scene?"

"I have a driver for the second rig and Prescott's on the way. You can respond directly to the scene."

"10–4. My ETA is about three minutes."

Ed and I have an unusual relationship. We've been

together for almost thirteen years, and he's the one who got me interested in ambulance work. Although we are lifetime partners he owns a house closer to the Prescott district and I own a condo near the center of town. Since we each work at home, we respond to ambulance calls frequently during the day and often meet at the scene.

As I turned onto Route 161, I saw that the police had the roadway blocked. The fire department had been called to the scene for logistical support and to wash gasoline off the roadway, if necessary. My flashing green light immediately identified me as a member of the ambulance corps, so the policeman waved me past the barricade. I parked about fifteen feet from the Jeep, which was now resting quietly against the tree. I grabbed a pair of latex gloves from my glove compartment and tried to pull them on over my still-sticky nails. My left middle finger stuck, leaving about an inch of glove finger extending from my hand. Shaking my head, I headed for the Jeep.

"What do you need me for?" I asked Linda, who was leaning over a supine figure on the ground. Tom was at the victim's head, holding one hand against either side of his face, keeping him from moving and doing more damage.

"This one's for the chopper. We're okay until we have more help. There are two more victims that way," she said, pointing farther down the road. "Do whatever you can."

"Will do, Linda." I saw two groups of people bent over what must be the two other victims. As I sorted out the bystanders and rescuers, I saw Heather Franks with one group, but at first glance there was no one I knew with the other group so I sprinted toward them.

As I arrived I realized that one crouched figure was Pete Williamson, wearing a white T-shirt with a bright EKG tracing across the chest and the words PARAMEDICS DO IT WITH RHYTHM in black letters. Pete is one of Fairfax's most experienced members, great to have on the crew in a difficult situation. A professional paramedic who's taken thousands of calls, his experience and calm demeanor are invaluable. Since Fairfax was only a basic life support organization and had no paramedic authorization, his greatest frustration was that, when he rode with Fairfax, he could function only as an EMT and couldn't do any invasive, and possibly life-saving, advanced life support procedures.

"Joan, glad you're here," he said, cutting the boy's shirt off. "Take over head stabilization and see what you can find out about this kid."

A bystander was crouched over the bloody victim, holding the boy's head. "Thanks," I said to the man in jeans shorts and a pink golf shirt. "I'll take his head now."

The man moved to one side and I placed one gloved palm against the left side of the boy's head, supporting him where he lay in the grass. "Don't move, okay? My name's Joan and that's Pete down there cutting your clothes so we can check you out. What's your name?"

"Joe. Joe Corelli. Am I going to die?"

"We're going to do everything in our power not to let that happen," I said. He looked awful, with blood smeared over his face and abrasions on all four extremities. "How old are you, Joe?" His answer would serve two purposes. First, I could assess his level of consciousness; second, I would know whether the hospital could treat him without needing to contact a parent or guardian.

"I'm eighteen," he answered.

"That's good. Do you remember the accident?" Another way to check his memory.

"Some asshole . . . cut us off. Then he slammed . . . his brakes." The boy was puffing, speaking in short bursts. A Fairfax police officer arrived with the oxygen cylinder from his trunk, hooked it to a non-rebreather facemask, and placed the mask over Joe's face.

"This will help you breathe," I told the young man. "Just try to relax and breathe gently. What hurts worst?"

"My side. I can't seem . . . to get my breath." His breathing was shallow but not too rapid, and his color was normal. So far so good.

"Does it hurt worse when you take a deep breath?" I asked.

"Yes," he said around the mask.

I saw Pete nod to me from Joe's feet. "Joe, wiggle your toes for me." Both Pete and I could see his toes move. "Any pain?"

"My legs hurt all over," he said, taking another breath, "but not worse when they move."

"Good." It's always best to keep only one person talking to the patient so, although Pete was clearly in charge, I continued talking to Joe. From all the other calls we had taken together I knew what Pete was doing and what he needed from our patient. "Pete's putting his hands against the soles of your feet. Press down like you were pressing on the gas pedal of the car." Pete nodded so I said, "Good. Now wiggle your fingers."

His fingers wiggled easily. "That's fine, Joe."

"Am I going to lose my leg? It really hurts bad."

"No, you're not going to lose anything that I can see." I looked over the boy's arms and legs and gave him a truthful assessment. "You're really bloody with road rash all over both arms and legs, but everything moves and works."

"Am I going to lose my ear?"

"Your ear?"

"It hurts and someone said it was all bloody."

"The one I can see is fine."

"It's the one that's on the grass right now."

Without moving his head, I slid one hand gingerly under his face and felt his ear. It seemed to be attached. I pulled my hand out and saw that, although it was bloody, the blood wasn't bright red.

"I don't feel or see any serious bleeding and everything feels attached. We need to roll you onto a board so we can get you on the stretcher and off to the hospital. We'll check it further then."

"Am I going to go to sleep?"

"Why would you think that? Are you bored?"

Joe gave me a look, then a tiny smile. "I'm sorry. I'm just scared."

"Of course you are," I told him. "That's natural. This isn't anything you've been through before."

"Get me to the hospital, please," he said, a bit louder.

"Joe, you have to be patient with us for a moment. Pete's got to finish checking you out."

An ambulance pulled up beside us with Marge Talbot driving and Sam Middleton in the shotgun seat. As they climbed out, Pete yelled, "Crash kit, board, head blocks, straps, then the stretcher."

"Okay," Marge yelled back.

"What's all that?" Joe asked, grabbing my arm.

"It's all right. Try to relax. We're getting a longboard and equipment to fasten you to it so we can move you safely. This is all standard precautions that we take with anyone who's been hurt like this." I tried to answer each of Joe's questions truthfully without frightening him further while Pete quickly got his pulse and respirations.

"What's he doing?" Joe said, squeezing my arm.

"He's got your wrist and he's checking your pulse. Then we'll take your blood pressure and bandage some of those abrasions."

"Abrasions? Is that serious?" Joe stared into my eyes, begging me to tell him that he wasn't seriously injured.

"Abrasions. Like scrapes. Have you ever fallen and scraped a knee, you know, where all the skin comes off?"

"Yeah," Joe said softly.

"Well, it's like that on several places on your legs and arms. Where were you in the car?"

"I was in the back."

"How did you get here?"

"I ran to get help."

"Good for you," I said. "And now the help is here." I watched Sam place a six-foot-long backboard on the ground beside Joe, then take quick measurement and remove the proper-size cervical collar from a blue canvas bag. He put the collar on the ground beside Joe so it would be ready when we needed it.

Pete finished taking Joe's blood pressure. "130 over 78," Pete said.

"Is that bad?" Joe moaned.

"Actually, that's very good. Your body's strong and doing just fine right now."

"You wouldn't lie to me, would you?"

Without letting go of Joe's head, I moved so I could look directly into his eyes. "No, Joe. Absolutely not. I won't lie to you."

Joe sighed. "Okay."

A policeman strode up to Marge and, after a brief conversation, she yelled, "I'm going to load the other patient. The first rig is transporting the kid down the road to the helicopter landing zone. That should be quick, so it will then come back for you." She climbed behind the wheel and moved her rig closer to her new patient.

"I want to go now!" Joe yelled. "I don't want to wait. Where's the ambulance going?"

Pete positioned himself behind the boy's back and snugged the backboard against his spine. "Happiness is going last," Pete said. "It means you're the least seriously injured."

"Really?"

"It means," Pete continued as he adjusted the placement of the backboard, "that others need to be transported more quickly than you do."

"Oh," Joe said.

"Pete," I said, "we need to check his right ear after we roll him. He says it's cut but I don't think there's any fresh bleeding."

"Sure, Joan," Pete said. "Let's lift his head easy, then I'll check his ear and we can collar him."

I slid my right hand under Joe's face, avoiding his injured ear, then lifted his head slowly until his neck was in line with his spine. Pete bent over and looked at Joe's ear. "Looks like a cut on the earlobe and some blood from a cut above your ear, but everything looks minor."

"Is it still attached?"

"It certainly is," Pete said. "You have everything you had before the accident."

"Are you sure?"

"We're sure," I said, trying to calm his fears.

Joe was quiet while Pete and Sam fastened the cervical collar around his neck to protect it from further injury. Then we log-rolled Joe onto the long backboard, moving his body as a unit, and used straps to secure him to it. We placed trauma dressings over his ear and used head blocks—yellow-plastic-covered five by five by ten-inch cubes of foam—to keep his head from moving on the board. 45–01 arrived with Linda Potemski driving, and she and Sam pulled the stretcher out of the back.

Suddenly Joe yelled, "We were all going to college next week. Mike wants to play basketball. He's dead, isn't he?'

"No one here worked on either of your friends so we don't know how they are doing. The driver—"

"That's Mike. I'm sure he's dead."

"Mike's going to the trauma center by helicopter so I'm sure he's not dead." I didn't say "not dead *yet*." "We're going there too, and I'll try to get someone to keep you informed of his condition when we get there."

"He's dead. I know it." Joe moaned.

I saw Linda preparing the stretcher for Joe's backboard. "Linda? How was the boy you transported to the chopper?"

"Don't really know," she yelled back. "We drove him to the LZ and turned him over to the flight nurses. Tom's going with them. I put the stretcher back into the rig and came back here."

"You heard?" I asked Joe.

"Yeah," Joe said. "Charlie was thrown out of the car. I saw him flying through the air. He's not going in the helicopter. Is he dead?"

"Joe, I'd tell you if I could. I promised that I wouldn't

lie to you so I won't say something that I don't really know about."

"Could you look for Charlie?"

"Charlie's in good hands," Linda said to Joe. "As I passed by before I saw several real good EMTs working on him."

"Please, go check," Joe said to me.

"I need to stay with you. I'll tell you everything I can find out when we get to he hospital. Okay?"

"I guess."

I saw 45–01 leave the scene. "Your friend Charlie is in our other ambulance, just leaving for the hospital."

"Joe, you weren't wearing your seat belt, were you?" Pete asked.

After a moment's hesitation, Joe said, "Sure I was. We always do."

Pete raised an eyebrow at me. Since the seat-belt law, we've seen a dramatic drop in the number and severity of injuries in auto accidents, but it also has caused people to lie about their use. I could tell from his expression that Pete shared my doubts about Joe's answer. He had trauma indicating that he probably had been bounced around inside the car, and he had no marks on his chest that might have come from the shoulder harness.

After we used wide tape to fasten the head blocks in place, we gathered around the backboard to lift the heavy boy onto the stretcher. "Move back, Joan," Pete said, mindful of my bad back. "We can handle this." Back problems are endemic in emergency medicine, usually caused by repeatedly lifting, crouching, and bending. I often lift, forgetting in the heat of the moment about my injured muscles. This time I gladly backed off, instead grabbing the oxygen cylinder.

"One, two, three," Pete called, as three firemen, a police officer, Sam, and Pete lifted Joe onto the stretcher, then into the ambulance. As we started our lights and siren run to St. Luke's Trauma Center, Pete and I got Joe's full name, birth date, and additional important information for the state report we fill out for every call.

Then we talked, trying to keep the boy calm. Other than responding to his increasingly agitated questions about his condition and that of his friends, most of the trip was uneventful.

I was at the post office picking up a piece of certified mail when the radio broadcast the first call for the ambulance. "That's your radio again, Ed," Sue, the postmistress, said. "It never seems to fail—it always goes off while you're in here. You going?"

I took my letter and quickly signed for it. "Yeah, I'll drive in that direction just in case. Thanks." I headed for my car and drove without any flashing lights, toward the parkway. As the radio reports got more urgent, I checked my light switches and flipped the one for my green light. Then I used my FVAC portable radio to let the police know I was responding. I've been an EMT for almost twenty-five years and I'm a member of both Fairfax Volunteer Ambulance Corps and Prescott's Fire Department Rescue Squad. Since in this state blue lights are for fire department use and green for ambulance personnel, I have to be very careful which light I use. Each service will take offense if I use the incorrect color light. This point might seem small to outsiders, but the sense of community within each organization is very strong.

I arrived at the scene and parked behind Joan's car. Then I switched off my light, pulled on a pair of gloves, and trotted toward the Jeep. The left-front fender was crushed and the passenger compartment was crunched where the driver must have been sitting. The swath of dirt on the roadway indicated to me that the rear wheels had remained spinning for several seconds after the impact. The car must have been really moving. All these facts help us in assessing injuries. From the "mechanism of injury" we can tell what problems are likely to occur. This looked like a bad one.

There was a crowd around a form on the ground. Recognizing Tom Franks and Linda Potemski working on the patient, I bent over. "What can I do to help?"

"Good to see you, Ed," Linda said. "We've got this one almost all packaged, and Joan's down there"—she pointed down the road—"with the second patient and Pete Williamson. Can you work with Heather on the third boy?" She pointed toward a small knot of people on the far side of the car.

"Sure." I walked briskly around the car and down the slight embankment toward a body lying in some deep grass. As I approached, I saw that the victim was a teenage boy who seemed to be unresponsive. Heather Franks was assessing his injuries while Bob Fiorella held head stabilization. The boy already had an oxygen mask over his face. "Glad you're here, Ed," Heather said. "Would you get a set of vitals?"

"Sure," I said. I looked down at the boy, who stared straight up, not making eye contact with anyone around. I took a blood pressure (BP) cuff and stethoscope from the crash kit on the ground beside Heather and fastened the cuff around the boy's upper right arm. "This is Ed," Bob said to the boy. "He's been with FVAC even longer than I have. Ed," he continued, "I'm told this is Charles Woo.

He was thrown from the car and isn't all with us right now."

The phrase "I'm told" said a lot. Our patient obviously wasn't able to tell Bob anything so the police had probably checked his wallet for ID. "Hi, Charles," I said, taking the young man's wrist and feeling for his radial pulse. Then, watching the sweep second hand on my watch, I counted the number of pulse beats in 15 seconds. Without moving, I then counted his respirations. I pumped the BP cuff, pressed the bell of my stethoscope against the flesh just above the crook of the boy's elbow, and began to release the pressure. I heard the first beat at 165 and the last at 95. "His pulse is 84, respirations 28, and BP 165 over 95," I said to Bob.

I pulled a ballpoint pen from my pocket and wrote the numbers on my forearm, just above the top of my glove. I used to write them on my glove, but often I tossed that glove into the red bag of medical waste before I remembered to record the vitals on the state-mandated PCR— prehospital care report. Now, when I don't have paper, I use my skin to make notes.

As I worked I listened to Bob trying to get the boy to respond to questions.

"Charles, can you hear me? Open your eyes."

Nothing.

"Charles," he yelled, "if you can hear me, move your hands."

The boy blinked and moved his eyes, but his hands remained still.

"He's not really responding but if I yell, he seems to hear me. He blinks and rolls his eyes." The boy blinked again, then just stared up into space. "His teeth were full of grass," Bob added, "so we assume he was thrown from the Jeep onto his face."

I looked at him. "He's lucky. There doesn't seem to be any serious facial damage."

"I suspect a bad tib-fib on the left," Heather said, "but I can't really assess it with his leg bent beneath him like it is."

"Want to straighten it?" I asked.

Heather nodded. "Can you help me?"

I moved around and grasped the boy's ankle and foot under his left buttock. Heather grasped his knee as a bystander supported his hips to keep them from moving any more than necessary. In one motion we untwisted his leg and placed it on the ground, as the young man screamed in pain.

Heather used her heavy shears to cut his jeans up the front. There was severe deformity midway between his knee and ankle but no break in the skin. His leg appeared to be broken. "Where's that rig?" Heather yelled.

"Just pulling up," someone answered.

"Okay," Heather said. "We'll get him on the board and splint his leg later. I don't want to wait. Ed," she continued, "get a collar." She held her fingers below Charlie's chin, then added, "I think a short." We use finger-widths to estimate the proper size of cervical collar.

Marge Talbot pulled the ambulance to a stop and together we got the collar, long backboard, and rest of the immobilization equipment. "Head injury, tib-fib, and I don't really know what else," I told her. "What do you know about the other victims?"

"I was with the third guy, the one Joan was with, and he seemed pretty good. Abrasions everywhere, a few more serious lacerations and rib pain, but he was conscious and alert and seemed stable."

"Know anything about the driver?"

"Nothing much. The chopper's on the ground so the flight nurses have got him now. That's about all I know."

"Okay."

We packaged Charles and loaded him into the ambulance. With lights flashing and siren sounding, Marge drove the patient, Heather, Bob, and me toward the trauma center. During the trip, Charles's condition seemed to improve a bit. About five minutes from the hospital, he made eye contact with me and asked, "What happened?"

"There was an accident," I said. Since he seemed to be reacting to me, I continued to ask questions. "What do you remember?"

"Nothing."

"Did you have breakfast?"

"Yeah. Mike, Joe, and I went to the diner. I remember that. Oh, God, my leg hurts so bad."

"I'm sure it does, Charles. We'll be at the hospital in about five minutes and they'll be able to give you something for the pain."

"Can't you give me something?"

"Sorry. We're EMTs here and we can't give any medicine. What's your full name?"

"Charlie Woo."

"Nice to meet you, Charlie. I'm Ed." I pointed out the other crew members. "That's Bob and that's Heather."

"Hi," Charlie said softly.

"Hi, Charlie," they both said.

"How old are you?" I asked.

"Nineteen."

"What hurts besides your leg?"

"I hurt all over. My neck. My face." He spit. "I've got junk in my mouth too."

"We know. You ate some grass when you landed."

"Landed?"

"We think you were thrown from the car."

"Car. Yeah. Hey," he said, putting the situation together in his mind. "Are Joe and Mike okay?"

"I don't really know," I answered. "They are both going to the trauma center, and we can find out there. Where in the car were you?"

"I was in the passenger seat. Mike was driving and Joe was in the back. Shit. This sucks."

"Yeah, it does."

We spent the remainder of the trip gathering additional information from Charlie.

When 45–01 was about five minutes from the trauma center, Pete said, "Hey, Joan, will you call this in? I want to get another set of vitals."

"Sure." I pressed the specific combination of numbered keys on the key pad to alert the trauma center to an incoming radio transmission. "Fairfax ambulance 45–01 to the trauma center."

"Trauma center on," I heard.

"Be advised we're en route to your location with an eighteen-year-old victim of a motor vehicle accident. Patient is conscious and alert, complaining of pain in his ribs on inspiration, numerous abrasions and lacerations." As Pete relayed a fresh set of vital signs to me, I told the hospital. "Pulse 72 and regular, BP 125 over 80, respirations 16 and shallow. Our ETA to your location is about five minutes."

"10–4, 45–01. Is this the patient from the auto accident on Route 161?"

"That's affirmative," I answered. "There are three victims in all, one coming by helicopter, one on 45–02, and this one."

"10–4, 45–01. We'll be awaiting your arrival. St. Luke's clear."

"45–01 clear." As I replaced the mike in its holder, Joe said, "Joan, I was in the hospital when I was six. I had my tonsils out. It was a small hospital down county and they were real nice. Can't I go there?"

"You're going to St. Luke's Trauma Center. It's best equipped to take care of you and your friends."

"Why? What's different about a trauma center?"

I suspected that Joe was asking questions to try to take his mind off the accident and the possible consequences to himself and his friends. I was only too glad to help. "St. Luke's Trauma Center is a hospital that specializes in caring for accident victims, people who have suffered trauma."

"What makes it a trauma center and not a hospital?"

"Well," I explained, "to be a level-one trauma center, a hospital has to have all types of doctors in the building at all times. They have everyone from pediatricians to neurosurgeons to take care of whatever emergencies arrive. If you needed your leg set, your appendix out, your burn tended to, or your baby born, they would be able to handle it." I watched Joe smile at the thought of him giving birth. "Okay, but you know what I mean."

"Is it a big place?"

"Do you really want to know all this?"

Joe reached out and took my hand. "Yeah," he said. "Please."

"Sure," I said, smiling. "St. Luke's actually used to be called the swamp since all of its buildings, old and new, are built on what used to be a huge marshland. It's in a town called Oakmont, and it's really a couple of dozen buildings of all ages. Actually a lot of it used to be an old school complex that taught teachers. That closed about fifty years ago and the hospital took over the buildings."

"So it's really old?"

"Yes and no. Some of the buildings are pretty old but they're used for clinics, for research, for teaching, and for the administrative staff. The biggest part of the main building where the ER is, is just ten years old, but it's connected to some of the old buildings with tunnels."

Pete, who was noting the latest set of vitals on the PCR, grinned. "To tell the truth," he said, "I've been lost in there several times, once while wheeling a patient to the burn unit. I think I ended up in the neonatal unit."

"Neonatal?" Joe asked.

"Newborn babies. They have an area that specializes in tiny babies who need special care. Those one- and two-pound, very early ones. They have a great success rate."

"You're not alone in getting lost," I said. "I was trying to take a wonderful little girl up to pedes and ended up in the cardiac cath area. That's where they work with people who have heart problems. They even do transplants here. It's really a great hospital."

"You won't get lost with me, will you? You'll get me to the right place, right?"

I squeezed Joe's hand. "We know right where the ER is. We come here several times a week."

"Mike came by helicopter, didn't he?"

"They have a landing pad just behind the ER so they can get patients right into the trauma rooms. By the time we get there they'll have him well taken care of." As I answered him, we pulled into the ambulance driveway and backed into the bay.

"Will you check on Mike for me? Please, Joan? And Charlie too."

"Of course I will, Joe. Let's just get you settled first." We opened the ambulance's back doors and lifted Joe's stretcher out. Sam, Pete, Marge, and I wheeled the boy down the long hall and into the trauma cubicle the nurse indicated. We transferred him to the gurney, and, almost immediately, Dr. Robert Englander, the attending physician, began examining Joe. Pete gave a quick report and detailed Joe's vital signs.

"If it's all right with you, I'll go find out about the other two victims," I said to the rest of my crew.

"Sure," Pete said. "I've got quite a bit to write and Linda and Sam can make up the stretcher."

I patted the back of Joe's hand and left the cubicle. I found Tom Franks in the hallway. "Hi," he said softly.

"Bad?"

"Yeah. Since there was room I came on the chopper with the flight nurses. It's not good." Tom described his experience so vividly it was as if I were there.

I arrived on the first rig and the scene was chaotic. It seemed there were victims everywhere. Will McAndrews, the first cop there, told me there were three.

"You sure there are only three?" I asked.

"Yes, I'm sure."

"Okay, radio in for us," I said, "and get the second rig here quick." I looked at the condition of the driver and added, "And tell them to launch the chopper. How are the other two victims?"

"I don't know yet."

I saw Pete Williamson's car pull up and watched him jump out. I couldn't have been happier to see anyone. "Pete, take the one about forty feet that way and Heather, the one over there. Linda, stay with me." Pete and Heather sprinted off while Linda and I headed for the Jeep.

The boy was still behind the wheel. The only impressions that I got was blond, tall, and real slim. The passenger compartment was crushed in from the left front and there was a deep depression in the windshield, obviously caused by the driver's head. The boy was covered with blood from several deep facial lacerations, and his right arm lay in his lap, with an open fracture. I could see the bone ends. He was completely unresponsive.

Linda put the trauma kit and oxygen duffel down, jumped into the back of the car, and quickly checked the boy's carotid pulse. "Pulse is rapid," she said, "and his breathing's quick and shallow." She took head stabilization and I grabbed for his left wrist. I couldn't get a pulse, so I knew that his blood pressure was very low. "Let's just quick board him out."

Will arrived at the side of the car. "The second rig's on the way and I've got several people en route to the scene. The helicopter had just arrived at St. Luke's with a burn patient from another hospital, did a hot off-load, and is back in the air. We set up the LZ in the middle school ball field. The fire department's handling that. What can I do?" As always, Will was great.

"Terrific," I said. "We'll take this kid to the landing zone in –01 then send it back to pick up one of the others. –02 can transport the third victim. We're a bit busy here. Will, can you get us a board, collars, and straps?"

"Sure."

I hooked up the oxygen and, as soon as we could, we collared the kid and moved him to the stretcher. I just had time to get a quick set of vitals. BP was low, pulse and breathing rapid. We loaded him into the rig and drove to the ball field.

The helicopter and the ambulance arrived at about the same time.

"The flight nurses were great," Tom said to me as we stood side by side, washing our hands. "They intubated him and started lines in both arms in no time. Man, they are good. So anyway, they said I could, so I came along in the chopper. I just wanted to be with the kid, I guess. I figured I could hitch a ride back on one of the rigs."

"Sure," I said as we walked together toward the major trauma room. "And I know what you mean about the flight nurses. They really are terrific. They've saved my patients' hash many times."

We arrived at the door of trauma 1 and looked inside at the unconscious figure of the driver, now fighting for his life. I counted seven scrub-suited figures around the stretcher, each working feverishly to do his or her task. One was cleaning the boy's groin area so they could start another IV line, one was adding medication to one of the existing IV bags, a third was attaching monitoring devices, and another was rhythmically squeezing the bag attached to the end of the tube in his trachea, forcing 100 percent oxygen into his lungs.

I caught the eye of one of the nurses. "I want to tell his friend how this boy is," I said quietly.

The nurse shook her head. "Severe head trauma. He's decerebrate."

"What's decerebrate?" Tom whispered to me.

As the nurse returned to other duties, I said, "Posturing. That means his brain is swelling and pressing on critical nerves and forcing his body into one of two possible positions, either fetallike or, like him, widely spread."

"He's not going to make it?"

"It's not good. I don't want to tell my kid that right now, but I can't lie to him either."

"I usually let the doctor do the telling," Tom said. "It seems to come better from someone they trust. And they seem to know how to do it."

I sought out Dr. Englander. "Doctor, how's Joe, the kid I brought in from the accident?"

"He'll be fine. He's in quite a bit of pain from the abrasions and I suspect a few broken ribs, but his vitals are strong. He seems like a tough kid."

"He's scared to death," I said, "but he's covering well. He wants to know about his friend, the driver, who's not doing well at all."

"I know. I was just about to tell him. Would you come with me? He seems to have developed a rapport with you."

"Sure," I said. Together we walked into Joe's cubicle.

From the look on my face, Joe must have known. "He's dead, isn't he?"

Dr. Englander said, "No. He's still alive, but it doesn't look good."

The change in Joe was immediate. "Oh, God! Oh, God! I want to see him. He'll be all right if I can see him. We're going to college in just a few days." His voice rose and he began to thrash. "I have to see Mike! I have to see him!" He ripped the just-established IV line from his arm and started to get up.

"Joe," I said. "You have to lie down. You can't help him this way."

"Joe," Dr. Englander said, placing an arm across the boy's chest, "lie down."

Suddenly Joe landed a punch to the doctor's jaw. "I have to get up. I have to see Mike."

Dr. Englander stepped back, rubbed his jaw, and said to a nurse who had entered when she heard the commotion, "I need some real help here."

"You want a Jupiter?"

The doctor nodded and the nurse went to the phone. I had heard of a Jupiter, a special alert for an unruly patient, but I had never seen one. "Joe," Dr. Englander said, "you're not helping your friend by acting like this."

Joe sat on the edge of the stretcher, putting on his shoes, with blood oozing from the site of the now-removed IV line and from several not-yet-bandaged abrasions and minor lacerations. "I gotta see him," he muttered.

In only a moment the first uniformed security guard arrived, quickly followed by three more. Joe jumped to his feet and tried to get past Dr. Englander, who now had sufficient help to wrestle him back onto the stretcher and strap him down.

As the doctor pushed me out of the cubicle, he said, "They'll take good care of him, you can rest assured. His parents are on their way, and Dr. Holbein is well trained to handle situations like this."

"Who's he?" I asked.

Dr. Englander indicated the white-jacketed man who was just arriving at a trot. "He's a psychiatrist with special training in grief counseling. There will be a priest too, if needed."

"That's good. Joe's a real nice kid."

"Of course he is. This is a difficult situation for anyone, much less a teenager who's probably never even considered death before. Facing one's own mortality is hard for any of us. Trust us. He'll be well taken care of."

"Thanks, Doc." As I walked out of Joe's cubicle, I saw Ed and his crew leave another. "I didn't realize you were here too," I said. "You must have transported the third kid. How was he?"

"He's actually doing well. His vitals are good and I think his injuries are probably minor. Yours?"

"Just terribly agitated. He really got to me. He's not badly hurt but he freaked when he was told that the driver's probably not going to make it."

"Shit."

"Yeah. Shit." I felt better just having Ed there to share the whole thing with. "They had to call a Jupiter."

"A Jupiter?"

I explained about the psych response I had just witnessed. Then I hesitated. "From the quiet, I assume he's calmer now." I saw a middle-aged woman talking to one of the nurses, then watched as she bustled toward Joe's cubicle. "Maybe that's his mom."

Ed and I hugged a lot the rest of the day, and I took another call. I guess it's like getting back on the horse.

I checked our local weekly paper the following week and read that the driver had died the night after the accident. Both Joe and Charlie had been kept overnight for observation, then released. Although Joe probably will not remember me at all, I'll remember him for a long time.

Chapter 3

Over the years, I've dealt with hundreds of children. They can be the most rewarding, the most frustrating, and the most heartbreaking of all patients. And I just love them all.

Eleven-year-old Barry Hayward woke up to the loud sounds of Hootie and the Blowfish one Wednesday morning. The clock-radio was extremely loud, but he and his mother had agreed that if Barry was going to wake up at all, the radio had to be set at a decibel level that would crack most people's eardrums. As he swam up toward consciousness, Barry realized that he really felt lousy. Since it was a school morning, his next thought was "Do I feel bad enough to get out of school today?" He lay in bed inventorying his body. Not nauseous, no sore throat—sore throats got you out of going to school really quick—no belly- or headache, nothing dramatic. He just felt yucky.

He reached over and turned the radio down, then slowly turned over and swung his legs over the side of the bed and tried to stand. Somehow, his legs wouldn't hold him up. As he sank to the floor, terrified, he screamed,

"Ma!" Barry swallowed hard, trying to stem the decidedly unmasculine tears that threatened to spill from his deep brown eyes.

Downstairs, Louise Hayward was just pouring Fruit Loops into a bowl when she heard Barry's scream. Unlike his frustrated or angry scream, this frightened yell caused Mrs. Hayward to drop the box on the floor and bolt up the stairs. As she entered Barry's ever-messy room, she found him in a heap on the floor, surrounded by piles of clean and dirty clothes. "Barry, baby, what's wrong? Did you fall? I've told you and told you to keep this floor picked up. And how can you tell the clean clothes from the dirty ones?"

"I didn't fall, Ma," Barry said. "I just can't stand up. My legs won't hold me."

Mrs. Hayward looked down at her son. An unusually healthy boy, Barry was big for his age, well muscled for an eleven-year-old, and extremely well coordinated. He played basketball, football, and baseball with the local kids, depending on the season, and was usually the best player on the team. He had medium-brown skin, a thick head of wiry hair that he had recently been trying to get into dreadlocks, and deep brown eyes that always seemed to find a joke in any situation. Now his eyes were swimming with unshed tears. "Okay, baby," Mrs. Hayward said. "Let's see whether I can help you up."

Although she was a slight woman, she managed to get Barry back into bed. As she watched him struggle to get toward the center of the mattress, she knew he wasn't moving right. Calming her rising panic, she sat on the edge of the bed. "Baby," she said, "I think we'd better call the doctor."

Although he was comforted by his mother's presence,

he found that his hands were shaking and he couldn't keep his heart from pounding. He took several deep breaths and tried to be brave. "Yeah, I guess," he said softly.

Mrs. Hayward pulled the sheet over her son's legs and tucked him in as she had when he was a toddler. Then she went into her bedroom, dropped onto the edge of the bed, took a deep breath, and picked up the phone.

Since it was not yet 8:00 A.M., when Mrs. Hayward dialed the pediatrician's office, she got his answering service. When she explained Barry's symptoms, the woman suggested that she not wait but call an ambulance. As frightened as her son, Mrs. Hayward dialed 911 and gave the dispatcher her son's symptoms.

"Mrs. Hayward," the dispatcher said, "we'll have an ambulance there in a few minutes. Is your house easy to locate?"

"It's the fourth on the left on Sycamore. There's a white mailbox and there's a basketball hoop on a pole beside the garage."

"Okay, they'll be there in just a short while." Both women hung up.

Next, Mrs. Hayward called her husband's office and told his secretary to have him call home as soon as he arrived. He had left before seven to drive into the city, and, unless traffic was extremely heavy, she assumed he would get there soon. As she put the phone into the cradle, she gathered all the internal strength she had and walked back toward her son's room.

Jill Tremonte, Fred Stevens, and I were the duty crew that morning. Fred, a great cook when he wanted to be, had just finished making a six-egg mushroom omelet, several pieces of toast, and a fresh pot of coffee when the call came in.

"Fairfax Police to Fairfax Ambulance."

"Shit," Fred said. "It never fails. First law of emergency medicine, don't ever plan to eat hot food. Joan, can you get that?"

"I've got it," Jill, crew chief for that morning shift, said as she grabbed the mike. "Fairfax on."

"The ambulance is needed at 1244 Sycamore, the Hayward residence, for an eleven-year-old boy feeling ill."

"10–4. 45–01 is responding to 1244 Sycamore for a boy feeling ill."

"10–4. Your time is oh seven five five."

We trotted into the garage. Fred climbed into the driver's seat and I got into the back. "I turned the stove off," he said before either of us could ask. Several years before Fred had left a frying pan on the stove and the fire department had had to be called. It was impossible to live something like that down.

Jill pressed the button to open the heavy garage door and, after Fred drove the rig outside, pressed the button to close the door. Then she climbed into the shotgun seat and, light flashing and siren wailing, we drove toward Sycamore.

"Probably a severe case of parentis panickus. Some frightened parent, all upset because little Johnny has a head cold," Jill said.

"Fairfax Police to 45–01."

Jill keyed the mike. "45–01 on."

"Be advised that it's the fourth house on the left with a white mailbox," the police dispatcher said.

"Thanks, and 10–4."

As we turned onto Sycamore, Jill and Fred spotted the white mailbox. Fred cut the siren and pulled into the driveway, just behind Fairfax Police car 305. Officer Chuck Harding was just walking up the front walk. While I grabbed the trauma kit, Jill and Fred followed the officer up to the front door.

They rang the bell and, as I walked up behind, we heard footsteps. The door opened and a frightened-looking slender black woman greeted us. "Thank God you're here. I'm so scared. Follow me upstairs."

"What seems to be the problem?" Jill asked, trying to hide her skepticism.

"He can't seem to walk or even stand up. I think he's paralyzed."

Suddenly Jill's expression changed. If this woman wasn't merely a bad reporter, this was a much more serious situation than just a panicky parent. "You're his mother?"

"Yes. Sorry. I'm Louise Hayward. My son's eleven and his name's Barry. He's always been such a healthy boy. Athletic, you know."

We arrived at the top of the stairs and walked into what was obviously a boy's room. The walls were filled with Boston team posters, the Celtics, the Red Sox, the Bruins. A huge image of Larry Byrd stared down at the desk. "Hi, Barry," Jill said, crouching beside the bed. "My name's Jill. What happened this morning?"

"I tried to get out of bed and I fell down. My legs didn't seem to hold me."

"Okay. Let's see." Jill slowly lowered the sheet that covered the lower half of the boy's body and saw that he was wearing a Celtics sweat suit. "You're sure a Boston fan," she said, uncovering the boy's feet.

"We just moved here last year from Chelsea," he said. "That's right near Boston. I'm still a fan but it's harder to see the games on TV now."

"I'll bet it is," Jill looked at the boy's toes. "Can you wiggle for me?"

"It's kinda hard. It feels all fuzzy."

She squeezed the big toe on his right foot. "Can you feel me?"

"Yeah," Barry said. She tried the other and got the same answer.

Jill placed one palm against the sole of each foot. "Press against my hands like they were bicycle pedals, Barry." She felt him push, but the response was very weak. Then she placed two fingers in each of his palms. "Squeeze." Those responses were a bit weaker than she might have expected, although not as weak as his lower extremities.

"Were you fine when you went to bed last night?"

"Yeah, I was great."

"Headache? Sore throat? Anything like that?"

"Nope. The rest of me feels okay."

"Well, Barry, I think we'd better get someone to look you over who knows more about boys and problems like this than I do."

His eyes wide, Barry nodded. "Yeah. I guess."

Earlier Fred had gone back downstairs, and now he arrived with the Reeves stretcher. "A stairchair would be easier, but I thought this might be better considering his weakness."

"I agree. Barry," Jill said, "these are my friends, Fred and Joan. They'll help me to get you into the ambulance."

His eyes still teary, Barry said, "I guess that means no school today."

Jill winked. "I'm afraid it does. Is that a great tragedy?"

For the first time, Barry's face looked a bit less grim. "Well, it's a great sacrifice, but I'll try to get over it."

"This is a Reeves stretcher," she told him, unrolling half a dozen six-foot-long slats held together with a gray plastic covering. "We're going to put you on this, then roll you up so we can carry you down your stairs. Okay?"

"I guess. Are you going to give me a shot?"

"Nope," Jill said. "No shots of any kind from any of us."

"But I see the paramedics give shots all the time on TV."

As Jill put a blanket on the Reeves to protect Barry from the cold plastic, I continued, "We're EMTs, Barry, not paramedics. We don't do some of the stuff that they do on TV."

"I thought you were all paramedics."

As Fred gently rolled Barry onto the Reeves I said, "Nope. An EMT goes to school for about one hundred hours."

"Yuck," Barry said.

"Well, we love what we do and go to school to learn to do it the best way we can. And we have to go back every three years."

"School after you're done? That's terrible."

"We don't really mind," Jill said.

Fred rolled the stretcher around Barry and fastened the straps. There was a space so the boy could see us all, but his body was completely supported. I grinned at Fred. "Well, most of us don't," I said, laughing. "Anyway, paramedics go to school for almost one thousand hours and learn how to give medicine and lots of stuff we can't do."

"Do you want to be a paramedic?" he asked me.

"Not really," I said. "I enjoy what I do as a volunteer. I don't want to make it my job, because if I *had* to do it I might not enjoy it as much. And to be a good paramedic you have to do it all the time to keep your skills up. It's like basketball. The more you practice, the better you get. I don't want to be a paramedic all the time. I like just volunteering a few times a week."

Fred, Jill, and I carried the Reeves down the stairs and, as we passed through the front door, the phone rang. "That will be my husband," Mrs. Hayward said. "He'll meet me at the hospital, so can I ride with you?"

"Sure," Fred said. "You can ride up front with me."

"But I want to ride with Barry."

Since Barry seemed comfortable with Jill and me, and, in general, relatives are better off in the front, Jill trotted out our usual excuse. "Our insurance forbids relatives from riding in the back, Mrs. Hayward," she said. "But I can assure you, Barry's fine with us." And just in case anything goes wrong, Jill thought, you won't be underfoot. Had she thought Barry would be better off with his mother in the back, she would have allowed it, of course.

"Where shall I tell my husband to meet us?"

Jill looked at me then said, "Trauma center?"

"I think so."

"Me too," she said as she turned to Mrs. Hayward. "Tell him to meet you at St. Luke's Trauma Center in Oakmont." Afraid that paralysis would spread to the boy's respiratory system, we wanted him in the most sophisticated local facility available. "They've got a great pediatrics unit." And a pediatric intensive care unit devoted to very sick children, I thought. Jill and I exchanged looks, both hoping that wouldn't be necessary.

Mrs. Hayward dashed into the house and returned a few minutes later.

In the ambulance, Jill took a quick set of vitals and, when Mrs. Hayward was buckled into the front passenger seat, we proceeded toward St. Luke's. Despite the rush-hour traffic on the parkway, it took only fifteen minutes to arrive at the ER.

Dr. Maria Sanchez was waiting in the hallway for the boy. As we wheeled Barry through the wide double doors and down the hall, Dr. Sanchez watched the deliberately cheerful faces of the crew. She was adept at reading expressions, and I knew she could tell that we were worried.

As she walked beside us, Jill said, "Hello, Dr. Sanchez. This is Barry. He has some weakness in his legs and reduced neurological responses in his upper extremities as well. He denies headache, sore throat, nausea, and he doesn't seem to have a fever. Pulses are good times four. Vitals are within normal range."

"Good," Dr. Sanchez said. "Let's get you into room 3 and we'll have a better look. Is a parent here with him?"

"His mother's in triage giving information. She'll be here in a moment."

We transferred Barry to the hospital stretcher and, with good wishes, left Barry in Dr. Sanchez's capable hands. As Jill was doing the paperwork, I eavesdropped on the doctor's conversation with Barry.

"Does it seem to be getting worse?" Dr. Sanchez asked Barry.

"Maybe. Just a little."

"That might just be the good news, Barry," Dr. Sanchez said. "I have an idea about what this might be. Do you play outside a lot?"

"Yeah. Almost every day."

"In wooded areas?"

"Sometimes. Is that important?"

"It might be. Do you have a dog?"

"No. Mom says we might get a puppy one day." While they talked, I could hear the rustling of the sheets, and I could picture Dr. Sanchez going over every inch of Barry's body with her hands. Barry giggled. "Hey, that tickles. What are you looking for?" he asked.

"I'll tell you only if I find it," she said. "But I haven't found anything yet."

I peeked through the opening in the curtains and watched Dr. Sanchez slip her gloved hands into Barry's hair, exploring his scalp with her sensitive fingertips. Suddenly she grinned. "There's a lump on your scalp in all this hair. Does this hurt?" she asked.

"Maybe just a bit. What is it?"

"I think it just might be a dog tick. It might be responsible for your problem." She stood up. "We're going to order blood tests and such, and we might have to shave a little of your fancy hair to see what's going on. If it is a tick, we can get this little beast out of you real quick."

"Will I get better?"

"I'm pretty sure you will." Just then Mrs. Hayward entered through the curtains, and Dr. Sanchez told her about the lump. "I think he has what's called tick paralysis. There's something in the tick's saliva that affects the nervous system. Once we get the beastie out, he should recover very quickly. We're going to run a few more tests, just to be sure, but I think that's the answer."

As we got back into the ambulance for the return trip to Fairfax, I shared what I had heard with Jill and Fred. "I read about a case of that about two years ago," Jill said. "Pretty scary."

I thought about my own two children and two grand-children and shuddered, knowing how I would have felt in a similar situation. "So they just get the tick out and he gets better?"

"Yeah, I think so," Jill replied. "From what I remember reading at the time, once the tick is removed the recovery is pretty dramatic. The paralysis can be gone in as little as a few hours."

"That's great," I said. I thought about my daughters' long blond hair. "They would have had just as much trouble finding a tick in my girls' hair as Dr. Sanchez had in Barry's. I'm just glad I never had to go through any-thing like that when my kids were young."

"Amen to that," Jill and Fred said simultaneously.

"Don't jump on the bed," Helen Donaldson yelled in the direction of her sons' bedroom. "Damn those kids," she muttered. "How many times do I have to tell them . . . ?"

The sounds continued and, about five minutes later, Helen pounded up the stairs. As she approached her sons' room, the thudding subsided. When she opened the door, her two darling boys, ages eight and six, were sitting like little angels, reading X-Men comic books. "Oh, hi, Mom," Greg, the older boy, said, glancing up and trying—but failing—to look innocent.

"Don't 'Hi, Mom' me. I have told you a thousand times that it's dangerous to jump on the bed. I won't tell you again. One more time and you're grounded. For life.

Do you understand?" She tapped her right toe on the rust-color carpet.

"Yes, Mom," Greg said, sighing deeply.

"Yes, Mom," his younger brother, Mark, repeated.

"And if I have to come up these stairs one more time . . ."

"We get the picture, Mom," Greg said, his eyes lowering to his comic book.

"Sorry, Mom," Mark said.

Mrs. Donaldson turned, left, and closed the door behind her.

As soon as the door closed, Greg dropped the comic book. "You've almost got it," he said to Mark. "Just a bit more spring and you'll be able to make a complete somersault."

"But Mom just told us not to jump any more."

"Mark, you have to understand mothers. They have to make speeches and tell us what to do. It's in the rules. But they never actually do anything about it."

"But we'll be grounded. No baseball, no scouts, no nothing."

"Oh, Mark, you're such a baby. How many times has she said that?" Greg looked at his younger brother and waited for an answer.

Mark thought seriously about Greg's question. "Lots, I guess," he said.

Greg stretched out on his back on the bed, crossed his legs at the ankles, and cradled his head on his stacked hands. "She threatens to ground us for everything. Like not cleaning the room, tracking dirt into the carpet, watching great scary movies on TV. She's said that zillions of times. Right?"

"Right," Mark said, stretching out on his bed and

arranging his body in exactly the same position as his brother. "Zillions of times."

"Okay. And how many times have we ever been grounded?"

Mark paused. "Well, there was that time when she found out we had put the glue in Linda McDougal's backpack."

"Yeah, there was that once. But other than that?"

Mark thought long and hard. "None."

"Right. Now are you going to learn that flip?"

"Sure, Greg. I can do it. I know I can."

"I know you can too," Greg said. "You just need a bit more bounce." Suddenly Greg jumped off the bed, pulled the blinds on the window beside Mark's bed up as high as they would go, then handed the cord to Mark. "Move toward the center of the bed so you don't fall and use this to give yourself a little pull. It should add just enough bounce."

"Yeah, Greg. Great idea." Mark held the Venetian blind cord in one hand and bounced several times, getting closer to the edge, but also getting a bit more height each time.

"Grab the cord closer to the top," Greg suggested.

Mark looped the cord in his hand and bounced one more time. As Greg watched, the cord became wrapped around Mark's neck and, on his next bounce, the six-year-old slipped off the edge of the bed, kicked two or three times, then ended up hanging by his neck, his still-wiggling feet only six inches off the floor.

"Mark, that's not funny."

Mark grabbed for the cord, struggled for a moment, then his body quickly went limp.

When his brother remained silent, Greg said again, "Hey, stop kidding around."

As he saw Mark's face starting to turn strange colors, Greg dashed across the room and tried to untangle the cord. "Mark. Get down. Stop this." The cord was knotted tightly and Greg's small fingers couldn't untangle it. He tried for what seemed like hours to remove the rope from around Mark's neck, but the more he tried, the tighter it became. He stepped back and stared at his little brother, the boy's face now blue. Suddenly paralyzed with fear, Greg stood still and, although his mouth moved, no sound came out. Finally a scream erupted.

In the laundry room in the basement, Helen Donaldson heard her son's shriek. She sprinted up two flights of stairs and, panting, opened the boys' door. For a second she remained rooted to the spot, then she crossed the room, lifted Mark's body and, without his weight to tighten the knots and tangles, quickly removed the cord from his neck. "Mark, are you okay?" She laid him on the bed then patted the side of his face. "Mark, baby, talk to me."

"I only wanted to help him do the flip," Greg whispered. "I only wanted to help him."

"Mark, don't kid with Mommy. Talk to me. Oh, God." She ran for the closest phone, the one in the guest room, and dialed 911.

"911. What is your emergency?" the operator's voice said calmly.

Mrs. Donaldson could barely speak. "I think my son's dead. He hanged himself. It was an accident."

"Is this the Donaldson residence at 1045 Franklin?"

"Yes. Hurry. He's dead."

"I'm getting the ambulance right now. Don't hang

up." Over the phone Mrs. Donaldson could hear the dispatcher talking to ambulance headquarters. She heard her address and the words "possible cardiac arrest."

The dispatcher returned to the phone. "How old's your son?"

"He's six."

"Is he breathing?"

Mrs. Donaldson's mind blurred. "I don't know. I need to get to him. Should I bring the phone into his room? Then you can tell me what to do."

"I'm sorry, madam, we don't give out any first aid information. The ambulance is on it's way. It'll be right there."

Helen Donaldson dropped the phone and ran back into her boy's room. Greg still stood in the same place and Mark still lay on the bed, unmoving.

At police headquarters, Mark Thomas dispatched cars 305 and 308 to the scene, knowing that both officers, as all the members of the Fairfax police force, were trained in CPR. "I hope they're in time," he said aloud.

As he heard police cars and the ambulance call in that they were on the way to a possible cardiac arrest, Officer Merve Berkowitz, who had been taking a break at headquarters, said, "I heard that call. I've always wondered how come we can't give out that over-the-phone CPR information like they do on TV."

"I tried to get authorization to do that," Mark said. "I asked the captain and took it to the town board. Everyone's worried about lawsuits. We would have to base our instructions on possibly inaccurate information given by bystanders. If they're wrong, or if they misinterpret or misunderstand what we tell them and someone dies or suffers some crippling complication, we might be held liable."

Merve shook his head in disbelief. "How many people won't benefit ..." Then he sighed and went back to reading the latest department memos on the bulletin board.

Pam Kovacs was unloading her dishwasher when the FVAC radio sounded the tones. "Fairfax Police to the ambulance corps." Pam noticed that the dispatcher sounded excited. Without waiting for an acknowledgment from headquarters, he continued, "The ambulance is needed at 1045 Franklin for a possible cardiac arrest."

Since Pam lived at 1055 Franklin, she grabbed her portable radio and sprinted out the front door. That's the Donaldsons, she thought, picturing the two small boys who made all the neighbors' lives difficult by riding their bicycles in the middle of the street and filling the mailboxes with toilet tissue at Halloween. She ran toward the house, up the front walk, and tried the door. Finding it locked, she leaned on the bell, then pounded on the door with her fist. She heard the door being unlocked and saw the older boy standing, looking dazed. Seemingly unable to say a word, he pointed toward the stairs.

Pam ran up the stairs and, hearing Helen Donaldson's voice, dashed toward the bedroom at the end of the hall.

"What happened?"

"I took him down." Mrs. Donaldson pointed numbly to the tangled blind cord. "He was hanging. I think he's dead."

Pam almost pushed the woman out of her way and knelt beside the bed, taking in the angry red line deeply grooved around the boy's neck. She leaned over close to the boy's face and pressed her fingers against the carotid artery in his neck. "No pulse, no breathing," she whispered. She pressed the SEND key on her radio. "45–12 to all units. Code 99." A confirmed cardiac arrest. "The patient's a boy age about seven. Expedite."

"He's only six," Mrs. Donaldson whispered.

Quickly Pam lifted the small body and placed him gently on the floor so she would have a firm surface on which to do CPR. She covered the boy's mouth with hers and gave two breaths. She watched as the boy's chest rose, glad that the rope hadn't crushed his larynx. Again she checked for a pulse and breathing and found nothing. "Go outside and wait for the ambulance," Pam told Helen. "Now."

"But—"

Pam got onto her knees and found her hand position for chest compressions. "Help them find the house as fast as they can. Now!" she told the woman, wanting her to help the rig find the house and also wanting her out of her way. As Helen left the room, Pam began compressions on the boy's small chest. "One, two, three, four, five." She gave a breath. "One, two, three, four, five." She gave another breath. Slowly she switched into autopilot, compressing, then giving breaths. After about a minute, she leaned over and again checked the boy's pulse and breathing. Surprised, she thought she felt a faint pulse. She checked again. The pulse was weak, but it was definitely there. "Thank you, God," she whispered. But the boy still wasn't breathing. She gave another breath, then one breath every four seconds, praying that the ambulance would arrive quickly.

I was on duty when the call came in for a boy not breathing. Although we respond quickly and efficiently to every call, when a child is involved, the heart pounds just a bit harder and the urge for speed is greater.

I jumped into the driver's seat of the ambulance with Sam Middleton riding shotgun and Steve Nesbitt in the back of the ambulance.

"Fairfax Police to unit responding to 1045 Franklin."

Sam took the mike from its holder. "45–01 on."

"Did you read that last transmission?"

"Negative."

"One of your members is at the scene. She states that it's a code 99. Boy of about seven."

"10–4. Our ETA is about three minutes." The squeal of the siren was urging other drivers to pull over, so we were making good time toward Franklin. "Don't push," Sam said softly, and I eased my foot on the gas just a bit.

"Sorry. It's hard not to press when it's a kid." We all knew that a speeding ambulance isn't immune to having an accident. I slowed to about five miles per hour at the red light at a major intersection and made sure that traffic all around me had stopped before proceeding.

Eventually I turned onto Franklin and saw both Chuck Harding's police car and a woman in jeans and a sweatshirt waving frantically. I pulled into the driveway and parked with Stan Poritzsky's car 308 right behind me. Sam grabbed the crash bag and defibrillator, while Steve got the long backboard we would need to carry the boy to the ambulance. Sam and I trotted into the house just behind the sweatshirted woman, with Steve right behind. "Upstairs," she said, panting.

As we ran up the stairs I saw a boy sitting on the floor at the top, looking like he was about to fall apart. As I approached, he said, "We were just playing. I didn't mean anything."

I patted his head as I passed. "We'll do everything we can and we all know it wasn't your fault." I try very hard to treat all the patients at a scene. Often family members are patients as much as the actual victim.

As we entered the small room at the end of the hall, I saw that Pam seemed to have the situation under control. She held a bag valve mask pressed against the small face and was rhythmically squeezing the bag, forcing pure oxygen into the boy's lungs.

"What happened?" Sam asked.

"Not sure," Pam said. "I found him on the bed. The mother's not really too coherent. She says he was hanging there," she said, motioning with her head toward the window.

Sam checked the boy's radial pulse and nodded. "Good pulse. Let's get him into the rig stat."

With Pam still bagging the boy, Steve and Sam positioned his still-limp body on the long backboard and strapped him down. While they worked, I felt I could spare a moment so I sat on the floor beside the older boy, who had followed me into the room. "Is that your brother?"

The boy nodded, large tears rolling down his face. "Is he dead?"

"No. His heart is beating and we're doing everything we can for him. What's his name?"

"Mark."

"And yours?"

"Greg."

"Well, mine's Joan. What happened, Greg?"

"Mom keeps telling us not to jump on the bed. I didn't know . . . He was jumping and got tangled. I didn't mean . . ."

I wrapped my arms around the small body and hugged him. As Steve and Sam passed me, I whispered in Mark's ear, "Accidents sometimes just happen. I'm sure it wasn't your fault. It wasn't your fault."

As the board reached the foot of the stairs, I heard Sam ask Mrs. Donaldson, "Are you going with us?"

"Oh, yes, of course."

"What about Greg?"

The woman looked at her son blankly. "I don't know. I can't leave him here alone. Can he come along too?"

Greg and I walked down the stairs hand in hand. "Sam. If you think Mrs.—?"

"Donaldson. Helen Donaldson."

"If you think she can ride in the back, I can take Greg here up front with me."

Sam stared at me. We had a bit of a problem. Having a relative ride in the back with a critical patient is usually a very bad idea. But Sam also understood that we needed to take care of Greg. Sam nodded, accepting the lesser of the two evils. "Mrs. Donaldson," he said, "you can ride in the back with us. I'll sit you in the crew chair and buckle you in." They maneuvered the backboard out the front door to where Chuck and Stan had already opened the wide back doors of the rig and opened the straps on the stretcher.

Pam continued to bag as she jumped into the back of the rig and Sam and Steve lifted the board onto the stretcher. As Sam climbed in behind Mrs. Donaldson, I heard him continue, "You will stay buckled no matter what. All right?"

"Yes. Of course," Mrs. Donaldson said.

I helped Greg into the passenger seat and checked that his seat belt was securely fastened. As I pulled out of the driveway toward Fairfax General, the closest hospital, I looked into my rearview mirror. An ambulance's rearview mirror allows the driver to see what's going on in the back of the rig, not the roadway. From the crew's body language, it looked as if things weren't going too badly. Since we were on a quiet, residential street, I turned off the siren.

"Hey, guys," I called. "Greg would like to know how his brother's doing. He's very worried."

"I know he's dead and I killed him," Greg muttered.

"Greg," Pam called, "Mark's doing better. He's breathing sometimes on his own and his color's good. I'm so glad you called for help as quickly as you did." Obviously Pam had picked up on my signals.

"Greg, baby," Mrs. Donaldson said, "you did just fine. Really." She reached through the walk-through and touched the boy on the arm.

"How old are you, Greg?" I asked. "You look about twelve."

Greg gave me a small smile. "No, I don't. I'm only eight."

"Oh," I said. "Got a girlfriend?"

"No. Girls are icky."

For the next few minutes Greg and I talked idly about school, teachers, and his friends.

"Hey, Greg," Pam said from the back. "Mark's breathing on his own. I think he's doing okay."

I hoped Pam was right, although we all knew that if his brain had been without oxygen for too long, serious brain damage might result. He wasn't out of the woods yet.

We got to the hospital and, while the crew unloaded Mark's stretcher, I helped Greg from the rig. Together we walked through the sliding doors to the ER. Mrs.

Donaldson knelt down and held her son close, then they both walked toward the admissions desk.

Fifteen minutes later, as we were about to leave, I saw Mrs. Donaldson and Greg walk into the cubicle where Mark was being treated. "Mom," said a small, hoarse but very much alive voice, "I didn't mean to jump on the bed."

Mrs. Donaldson began to cry and I heard Greg say, "It's okay, Mom. It's really okay, Mark. You know, accidents sometimes just happen."

"Sounds like he'll be okay," I said as the four of us walked out toward the ambulance.

"Yeah," Pam said. "Dr. Margolis said that he seems to remember everything. He'll probably have no lasting aftereffects."

I held my hand up to high-five Pam. "You did it," I exclaimed.

"Damn straight," she said, slapping the hands of all the crew members. "Damn straight I did. *We* did."

"Fairfax Police to the ambulance corps," my radio squawked. Good Lord, I thought, another call. Two of our ambulances were already out. It was a midwinter Sunday, and the recent blizzard had been over for two days. The sun was shining brightly. During a heavy snow, our call volume usually drops. People stay home, stay quiet, and don't usually get into trouble. But when the snow stops . . . Today the ambulance had responded for a person with chest pains while shoveling snow and a man who had fallen off his roof. He probably had been up there lightening the snow load.

When there was no answer from headquarters, the police set off the pager tones. "Fairfax Police to all home units. A full crew is needed for a sledding accident on the hill next to the high school. Any available units please call in." I had a pot of stew simmering on the back of the stove and was expecting a phone call so I waited, hoping that, on a Sunday, others would be available.

"45–75 will pick up the rig," I heard Jill Tremonte's voice answer.

"10–4, 45–75."

"45–52 will respond as an attendant." That was Tim Babbett, a new probationary member who was not an EMT or qualified to drive the ambulance yet.

The tones sounded again. "Fairfax Police to all home units. A driver or an EMT is still needed for a sledding accident. Be advised the patient has been moved to the front of the high school."

"10–4," Jill said. "I will be responding with 45–03 in one minute. Member Babbett is with me. Have you anyone else yet?"

"Negative," Mark Thomas said.

After deciding to let the answering machine take my phone call, I turned off the stove, pulled on my coat, and pressed the SEND key on my portable radio. "45–24 to Fairfax Police."

"Police on."

"I will respond directly to the scene as an EMT or driver."

"10–4, Joan. All units be advised the call is covered."

As I drove toward the high school, I thought about the possible consequences of a sledding accident. Broken necks are common, I thought, but if the patient had been moved to the front of the high school, I assumed that the injury was far less serious.

As I approached the high school entrance, I watched

the ambulance, light flashing, pull out and turn toward Fairfax General. "45–24 to 45–03. Do you still need me?" Maybe someone showed up unexpectedly and they had a full crew.

"Yes," a voice said. Then the rig pulled to the left shoulder of Route 10 beside the sledding hill and stopped facing traffic, lights still flashing.

"I can't stop here," I muttered. Due to the mounds of deep snow, there was insufficient shoulder on either side for safe parking. I couldn't see the driver's side door of the rig, but there was a police officer running across the field toward the base of the hill about forty yards away. Frustrated and totally confused, I pulled into the next side street and parked my car. Then I ran to Route 10 and crossed during a break in traffic. I looked toward the base of the hill and saw that a small crowd had gathered. They weren't at the high school after all, I realized. I looked at the officer's footprints through the snow and climbed up the deep pile of plowed, hard-packed snow and over the guard rail.

Suddenly I was up to my knees. Damn, I thought, there's no crust. The officer's footprints were significantly deeper than I had realized, but now I was committed. As I slogged on, my boots filled with snow and I had to lift my legs to almost hip height with each step. The officer's stride was considerably longer than mine, so I was forced to forge my own path. After what seemed like hours but was really only a few minutes I was halfway across the snow, struggling to get my breath. I stopped, panting, and looked at the cluster of people. I recognized Jill, Tim, and Officer Will McAndrews working on someone lying on the ground assisted by a crouched figure in a bright orange, one-piece ski suit.

I was panting and my heart was pounding when I finally reached the patient. Jill had done a good job of fully and tightly immobilizing the woman and securing her to a longboard. Nick Abrams, wearing an international-orange ski suit, was helping.

"Hi, Joan," Jill said. "Mrs. Davis was sledding on one of those inner tube things and fell out halfway down the hill. She slid the rest of the way on her shoulder and back."

"How did you guys get here?" I asked Jill and Tim, hoping there was an easier way than the one I had taken.

"We came in from the high school side, then skidded down the hill."

"Can we toboggan her back up the hill?" I asked.

"We can't find anything wide enough to guarantee her a safe ride," Jill said. "I think we've got enough man-power. We'll have to carry back the way you and Will came in." I looked at the two paths Will and I had made from the roadway to the foot of the hill and knew that I couldn't make it again.

"I can help carry," Nick said, "but I can't go to the hospital with you. I was here with my daughter when I saw the accident. Hey, Joan! You okay?"

"I'm all right," I replied, puffing.

He looked around. "Listen. We've got enough people. We can manage her." He indicated the trauma bag and the collar bag. "You just take those."

Jill, Nick, and Tim, assisted by Officer McAndrews and three bystanders, lifted the longboard and started through the knee-deep snow toward the ambulance. Without protest about how I could carry too—at fifty-four I'm getting too old for the heavy work—I lifted the bags. Deciding that up the hill was easier than through the snow again, I skidded and slipped my way uphill, down the narrow pathway toward the high school, and along Route 10 toward the ambulance.

I arrived almost at the same time as the group carrying Mrs. Davis. As I caught my breath, the injured woman was lifted onto the stretcher and into the rig. I climbed into the back with Tim to help until it was time to drive. Jill stayed outside to gather information from the woman's friends.

Tim reached for a pair of EMT shears and held the cuff of the woman's left jacket sleeve. "Don't do that yet," I said.

"Why not?" Tim asked. "We need to look for possible shoulder injury. She's complaining . . ." He again started to cut the jacket sleeve.

"Don't cut yet," I said again. "It's a down jacket."

"And . . . ?"

"If you cut that, we'll have feathers all over the inside of the rig. Let's wait a moment and see if there's another way, ma'am," I said, "where does it hurt?"

"My left shoulder. Real bad. My arm won't move right."

"Did you fall on that side?" I asked.

"Stupid inner tube just threw me out onto that shoulder. My fingers tingle too."

"Is this a down jacket?" I asked.

"I heard what you told this nice young man, but I'm afraid it is down. I can try to take it off—"

"No, you can't," I said quickly. "We'll do what we have to do to keep you safe." I got a roll of wide, silver duct tape from the cabinet and opened the straps that held the woman to the backboard. "Okay, Tim," I said. "You cut as close to the seams as you can and I'll try to tape up the cuts."

As Tim snipped and I taped, I gathered information from the victim. "I'm fifty-seven," she said. I raised an eyebrow. "I know," she continued. "I'm too old for sledding, but my grandchildren dared me."

I smiled. "I know just how that is. I have two grandchildren myself and I would probably do anything for them also. Besides your shoulder and arm, does anything else hurt?"

"No."

Tim continued to cut and I taped. Despite our efforts, the floor of the rig was becoming littered with feathers.

"Can you wiggle your toes?" I watched her feet move. "And your right hand, can you move the fingers?" She did so without trouble. "Now try the fingers on your left hand, but don't do anything that causes pain." Slowly, experimentally, she moved her fingers.

"They move okay," the woman said.

"Great." Tim and I had gotten the seam of the jacket cut from wrist to neck. As Jill climbed into the rig, I palpated Mrs. Davis's neck around the collar, her shoulder, arm, and chest. "I think this might be dislocated," I said, "but they'll need X rays to confirm that."

Jill took a quick set of vitals—they were all within the normal range—and, in only a few minutes, we were ready to go. I moved to the driver's seat and proceeded, code 2, toward Fairfax General Hospital.

After I backed the rig into the ambulance bay, I walked around to the back. As I opened the double doors, I was enveloped in a cloud of tiny feathers. The floor of the rig was about an inch deep in down. My taping job hadn't been of much help. We pulled the stretcher out and, trailing puffs of down, wheeled Mrs. Davis into the ER.

"Room 1," one of the nurses said, and we quickly transferred our patient to the hospital gurney. Dr. Frank Margolis examined her as I made up the stretcher and Jill completed the paperwork.

"I think this is just a dislocation," the doctor said, "but we'll do an X ray just to be sure. Unless something is very different from what I suspect, you'll be out of here in a few hours."

"That's great, Doctor," Mrs. Davis said.

I heard Dr. Margolis sneeze and Mrs. Davis say, "God bless you."

Dr. Margolis walked slowly from the trauma room, a small cloud of feathers trailing behind him. "Mary," he said to one of the nurses, "get housekeeping down here stat. Get that stuff"—he pointed to the feathers—"cleaned up. Now!" He sneezed again.

Jill and I giggled as we wheeled the freshly made stretcher toward the ambulance. Suddenly a cloud of feathers flew from the back of the rig. As we approached, we saw Tim, a piece of cardboard in his hand, trying to brush the down out the back door. Some landed on the ground but almost as much floated, then ended up back in the ambulance. Laughing, Jill and I wet several small towels and slapped at the feathers with them. As the down became damp, Tim was able to brush it out the door.

Thirty minutes later we were on our way back to the scene so I could pick up my car. "Never again," Tim said. "Never again will I cut a down jacket. Never again."

"I hope that's true," Jill said. "This is my third time."

"Oh," Tim said. "But what if there had been blood?"

"Oh, well," Jill and I said in unison. "You do what you have to do."

Chapter 4

Although we are sometimes treated as heroes, in our combined thirty-five years in the emergency medical services, Joan and I have seen very few instances of true heroics among EMTs. Sometimes we do save lives; when we do, we receive awards and often newspaper articles extol our heroism, even though all we did was perform CPR and defibrillation, skills for which we are well trained. For me the great feelings I have when I have been on a crew that has saved someone's life have nothing to do with awards or praise for heroism. Saving a life is its own reward, and it's a great one.

What seems closer to heroism to me are the times when EMTs struggle to save a life knowing that there is little or no chance they will be successful. We work as hard as we can despite our feelings of helplessness. When we fail, no matter how valiantly we have tried, there are no awards and there is no praise, except from each other.

As EMTs, Joan and I rarely, if ever, face personal danger. The ultimate in heroism, in my opinion, is when an EMT, or anyone else, risks his or her health or jeopardizes his or her personal safety to try to save someone's life.

* * *

Eighty-five-year-old Sy Weinberg had an appointment with his doctor. Despite his advanced age, Sy was in excellent health. His enlarged prostate had been giving him some problems, but his doctor had told him that he probably would not need surgery. Still, it needed to be checked every six months or so.

It was a cold, mid-November morning and a light coating of snow had fallen during the night. As Sy approached his car, he thought that perhaps he should walk to Dr. Connally's office. Since the office was in Hamilton Village, the retirement complex where Sy lived, and only a quarter mile away, it would be good exercise. Although Sy prided himself on walking at least a mile every day, this morning the ground was slippery and, besides, if he walked, he would be late. Sy opened the trunk of his car, took out a brush, and carefully cleaned all the snow from the windshield. After putting the brush back in the trunk, Sy got into the car, started the engine, and drove the short distance to the doctor's office.

Only moments after leaving home, Sy pulled into a parking space next to the medical building in the section that faced a small pond. He stopped for a moment to admire the frosty landscape and gaze at the small body of water that was ringed with a thin film of ice. After shifting into "park," Sy reached over to turn off the ignition but accidentally knocked the shift lever into "drive." The engine, which had not had enough time to warm up, was racing, and as the gears engaged, the car lurched forward. Startled and shaken, Sly slammed his foot on what he thought was the brake but hit the gas pedal instead. The car flew forward and bounced over the curb and down the shallow, snow-covered embankment into the pond.

Sy felt the bumping stop as the car hit the water and began to float away from the shore. Not realizing that the car was now in the water, Sy tried vainly to drive out of the pond. Within a few seconds, however, icy water began to fill the bottom of the car.

In a panic, Sy tried to open the door. The pressure of the rising water prevented him from doing so. The last thing Sy saw as the water rose around him was the face of Lynn, Dr. Connally's receptionist, staring at him in horror through the office window as he frantically banged at the car window with his fists.

Jim Masterson, one of FVAC's newer EMTs, had stopped at headquarters to restock his crash kit. The previous evening he had been the first EMT at the scene of a personal injury automobile accident, and he had used 4 × 4s (gauze squares), several rolls of gauze, and some tape. Like most Fairfax EMTs, Jim carried a fully stocked first-aid crash kit in the trunk of his car, and he liked to be sure it was complete. He had just finished counting out the proper number of gauze pads when the klaxon sounded.

"Fairfax Police to the ambulance corps." The sound of Mark Thomas's voice told Jim that the call was serious.

"Go ahead," Greg Horvath said. Fairfax's part-time dispatcher was in the kitchen, out of Jim's sight.

"Dispatch the ambulance to the pond behind the medical complex in Hamilton Village. We have a report of a car into the water with someone trapped inside."

"10–4. I'll be paging out for a crew."

"Be advised that the fire department's en route."

"10–4."

As Jim dashed into the kitchen, Greg said, "I heard Mike DeVito's voice. The fire engine's already en route. Can you go?"

"Sure," Jim said. "I'll respond with the rig. Page out for a crew to meet me at the scene."

"You got it," Mark replied.

Jim ran to the front of the ambulance bay and pushed the door button, unplugged the electrical charging line from the ambulance, climbed in, and started the engine. As the bay door rolled up, he switched on his emergency lights and, siren wailing, rolled toward Hamilton Village.

"GKL–642 Fairfax to all units," Mark's voice said. "The ambulance is responding to the pond behind the medical building in Hamilton Village for a person reportedly trapped in a submerged vehicle. A driver or EMT and an attendant are needed to meet the ambulance at the scene."

As Jim drove, he prayed for manpower. This sounded like a bad one.

He pulled the ambulance alongside Engine 44–31, facing the pond. He could see only the roof of the submerged car, about twenty feet from shore. A cable ran from 44–31's winch into the water. Mike DeVito was standing in front of the engine, struggling with the two levers that control the winch. He was dripping wet from head to toe. "I got the car hooked," he shouted as Jim got out of the ambulance, "but the damned winch is jammed. I can't pull it in. I tried to go down into the car but the water was so muddy I couldn't see a damned thing."

"Keep working on it," Jim said. "We've got to get the car into shallow water."

Jim knew that, although under normal conditions a

person could not survive without oxygen for more than four to six minutes, cold-water drowning victims had been successfully resuscitated with no brain damage after as long as three-quarters of an hour underwater.

For a moment he hesitated, looking at the ice-rimmed pond. Then he threw off his ski jacket, pulled off his work boots, and plunged head first into the frigid water. Half wading and half swimming, he made his way to the car, its roof about a foot below the water's surface. As he ran his hand down from the roof, he realized that the driver had been able to get the side window open but obviously hadn't been able to get out. Resting for a few seconds with his feet on the window ledge, Jim filled his lungs with air then dove in through the window.

Below the sparkling surface, the water was so murky that Jim could see only a few inches in front of himself. After grabbing the steering wheel, he pulled himself into the vehicle and along the length of the driver's seat. Feeling nothing, he turned and groped along the floor of the driver's side of the car and under the dashboard. He neither felt nor saw anything.

Breath exhausted, Jim returned to the surface and rested for a few moments, filling his lungs with air. The guy must be in the back, he reasoned. Despite his shivering, he dove toward the submerged car again. The rear window was closed. Frustrated, Jim went through the front window again and tried to get to the rear of the car. His passage to the backseat was blocked by the car's high headrests. He looked over and between them but could see nothing, so he reached through the opening and groped along as much of the rear floor as he could reach. Still nothing.

When he returned to the surface again, Jim needed

more time to catch his breath. His hands were beginning to get numb from the cold and his eyes burned from the gasoline that was rising from the vehicle and accumulating on the surface.

By that time Fairfax EMT Phil Ortiz had arrived, stripped off his coat and shoes, and made his way out to where Jim was standing, supported on the driver's window ledge. He had a crowbar in his hand. "The engine driver's still trying to get the winch to work, but he gave me this. I thought we'd need it." He peered into the almost opaque water. "I'll go down this time."

"No. I know my way around down there. I'll go back in just a second." Jim grabbed the heavy steel bar with fingertips already blue from the cold. "I must have missed the body when I checked the passenger front. I'll try that side again."

"Could he be in the back?"

"I don't think so," Jim said, taking a few more deep breaths. "I can't get around the headrests so I don't think the body could have either." Jim climbed up on the roof of the car and, leaning over the passenger side, smashed the front passenger-side window. "Phil, stay on top of the car in case I run into trouble." Then he dove into the car again. He explored the front passenger side, hoping he had missed something the first time, but he could find nothing except a shirt and a Styrofoam cup that floated at the vehicle's ceiling. When he surfaced again, Jim was starting to feel tired, but all he could think of was the fact that time was going by and someone was somewhere in the car.

Jim dove into the car for the fourth time. This time he tried to make his way past the front seats and headrests. While he might have been able to squeeze himself into the back, he wasn't sure that he would be able to get back out. His hands were now almost completely numb, he was starting to feel weak, and his lungs felt as if they were about to burst. He knew he was running the risk of becoming a victim himself.

When he surfaced, Phil grabbed his shoulder and said, "You look terrible. Let's get you back to shore." Reluctantly Jim nodded.

With Phil's help, Jim started toward shore, unaware of the blood that was flowing into the water from his numb arm, which he had lacerated on the broken car window. Barely able to stand even when they reached shallow water, Jim gratefully wrapped his uninjured arm around Phil's neck.

By now Fairfax Police Officer Merve Berkowitz had arrived. He splashed knee deep into the icy water and helped Jim out of the pond. While Phil turned and went back out to the submerged vehicle, Merve helped Jim walk unsteadily to the ambulance. Together they squeezed as much of the water out of his dripping jeans as they could. "You're staying here," Merve said, pushing Jim into the warm ambulance. "Your hands are blue and may be frostbitten and you're too damn cold. You need to be seen at the hospital when we transport the victim." Then he climbed in and bandaged Jim's lacerated arm. "Sit here and warm up," Merve ordered, then he climbed back out and walked toward the crowd gathering at the edge of the pond.

After Phil had gotten Jim to shore, he made his way back to the car, wading where he could, dog-paddling where the water was deeper. When he arrived at the submerged vehicle, he rested his feet on the window ledge and stopped to catch his breath. Suddenly he felt the vehicle jerk and slowly begin to move as 44–31's winch gears finally engaged. He held onto the roof as the car was slowly dragged toward shore. As the rear window began to emerge, Phil leaned over and peered into what was now revealed as a hatchback. As the water level fell, Phil saw a large object pressed against the hatch window—the body of a man. "I see him," he shouted.

Two police officers and three firefighters waded out to the car while Phil grabbed the crowbar and smashed the hatch window. Within a short time, Sy Weinberg had been removed from the car and carried to the shore.

As Phil slogged out of the pond and started toward the ambulance crew, Merve Berkowitz grabbed his arm. "What do you think you're doing?" he asked.

"I need to hook up the cardiac monitor," Phil answered, dripping and shivering.

"You're hypothermic yourself," Merve said. "Get into my car and warm up. NOW!" he ordered, leading Phil toward the patrol car, its heater blasting. "We have another ambulance responding to transport you to the hospital."

"Me? I'm really okay."

"You're shivering all over, your lips are blue, and you're unsteady on your feet. Now move."

"Yes, sir," Phil replied meekly.

Bob Fiorella and Heather Franks had arrived almost simultaneously in response to the dispatcher's call for help. As Sy Weinberg's body was being carried from the water, they assembled the equipment they would use to try to resuscitate him. Three firemen lay the soaking body on a backboard, and, while Bob routinely checked pulse and breathing, Heather used heavy shears to remove the man's sopping clothing. Then she used several towels and blankets to dry him off so they could get a reading with the defibrillator, the machine that had saved many other lives.

"No pulse," Bob said, combining forces with recently arrived Tim Babbett to do CPR. As the two worked with a bag mask and chest compressions, Heather placed the large shocking electrodes on Sy's chest—the red lead on his left rib cage, the white on his right upper chest. Then she opened the defibrillator and said, "Stop CPR." She gazed at the screen, hoping for some cardiac activity. "He's flatline," she said. Since there was no electrical activity in the heart muscle, the semiautomatic defibrillator wouldn't allow a shock to be delivered to Sy's cold, blue lifeless body.

In cases of cold-water drowning, a person is not considered dead until he's warm and dead, and Sy was certainly not warm. His blue-tinged skin felt almost as cold as the icy water in which he had been submerged for almost half an hour. The crew knew that, although people had been revived after being submerged for longer periods in cold water, the survivors always were young. And Sy certainly wasn't young. Although the crew couldn't use the defibrillator to "jump start" the man's heart, they would do CPR and transport him to the hospital.

With the help of the police and firefighters, Sy was loaded into the ambulance, where Jim was sitting, still shivering despite the warmth of the heater. Bob quickly hooked up the BVM to the onboard oxygen, placed the mask over Sy's face, and began ventilating him while Tim did chest compressions. Heather continued to dry Sy's body and remove the remainder of his soaked clothing. Not realizing that Jim had been in the water, Bob looked up at him and said, "Okay, Jim, let's go. Code 3."

Most of the feeling had returned to Jim's fingers and he was no longer as exhausted as he had been earlier, but he was still cold and his lower body was still in his original wet clothing. "Isn't Phil supposed to be the driver?" he asked Heather.

"I don't know who's supposed to be the driver," Bob snapped as he squeezed the BVM. "All I know is that Phil is hypothermic. He's in Merve Berkowitz's patrol car waiting for another rig to come and transport him. You're here so you drive."

"Okay," Jim said. He got behind the wheel, switched on the siren, and began to roll toward the closest hospital, Fairfax General.

Having been alerted to the arrival of a cold-water drowning victim, a trauma team was ready and waiting when the FVAC ambulance arrived at Fairfax General four minutes later. Two doctors, several nurses, and a number of support personnel worked in the trauma room, knowing that it was going to be of no use. They checked for heart activity, administered a small group of drugs, and shocked his heart, hoping for any sign of electrical activity. They used heated blankets and chemical heat packs to warm Sy's body. Despite their efforts, however, twenty minutes later they "called the code" and ceased their efforts.

After transferring their patient to the care of the emergency room staff, Tim, Bob, and Heather began to collect their equipment and replace their disposable materials. They didn't notice that Jim was quietly sitting in a chair, shivering and staring into space. As Rosemary Harper, one of the emergency room nurses not involved in Sy Weinberg's care, walked past, she suddenly stopped. She placed the palm of her hand against Jim's icy cheek. "Were you in the water too?" she asked Jim. "You're frozen."

"Yeah," Jim replied. Now that the adrenaline had completely worn off, he felt dazed and a bit disoriented. "Merve gave me his jacket."

The crew instantly stopped what they were doing and looked at Jim. They hadn't known that he had been involved in the rescue and, focused as they had been on their patient, they had never noticed that much of Jim's clothing was soaked and that he was trembling. Horrified, they realized that he was probably hypothermic and in need of medical treatment himself.

Bob, Heather, and Tim rushed to Jim's side and, with Rosemary's help, led Jim to a gurney in an available bay. "Tim, Bob, we're a bit shorthanded," Rosemary said. "Can you give us a hand and get all of those wet clothes off?" When they agreed, she drew the curtain and bustled away. As she returned with an armful of warmed blankets, the emergency room radio began to buzz. "Fairfax Ambulance 45–02 to Fairfax General Emergency."

Patty Stewart, one of the youngest ER nurses, walked over to the radio console and pushed the RECEIVE button. "Go ahead, 45–02."

"Be advised we're en route to your location with a twenty-one-year-old male hypothermia victim. His pulse is 80, respirations 24, BP 125 over 75. He is alert and oriented times three but he is shivering violently. Our ETA is three minutes."

"10–4, 45–02. Room assignment on arrival. Fairfax ER clear."

"45–02 clear."

"That must be Phil," Heather said from where she was putting fresh linen on the stretcher.

"Was he in the water too?" Patty asked. For the past several weeks Phil had been flirting with Patty every time he brought a patient to the ER. She was sure that he wanted to ask her out and had been wondering how to make it easier for him. "I'll go over to the ambulance entrance and meet the rig," she said casually. "In case they need some help."

A few minutes later, Patty watched the ambulance back toward the emergency room doors. As the crew unloaded the stretcher, Patty approached Phil who lay under a mound of blankets and a yellow thermal cover. "Well, look who's here," she said, pretending to be surprised.

"H-hi," Phil answered sheepishly, somewhat embarrassed but also delighted at being Patty's patient.

"Didn't your mother ever tell you not to go swimming in November?" she admonished.

"H-how else could I g-get a pretty n-nurse like you to t-take care of me?" Phil said.

Patty helped wheel Phil into the bay next to the one where Jim was being treated. "Get your clothes off," Patty said as she pulled the curtains around him. "Much as I'd enjoy helping you with that, I think I'll get one of the guys to assist."

"Yeah," Jim called from the adjoining bay. "It's real embarrassing being stripped by people you know."

"But don't go away, Phil," Patty said, her voice almost crooning. "You're going to see a lot of me over the next few hours. From what I hear, you and Jim are real heroes. So I'm going to take real good care of you."

"Phew," Jim said. "I wish she'd say that about me."

"Eat your heart out," Phil said. "Us heroes require lots of tender loving care."

Sy Weinberg was pronounced dead at 10:14 A.M., only sixty-two minutes after his car went into the pond. Jim required seven stitches to repair the laceration on his arm. He was admitted for observation and released the following day. Phil was treated and released the same day. He and Patty began dating a few days later. A small article about the incident appeared in the local paper the next day. The facts were mostly incorrect, and none of the rescuers received any recognition for their efforts—except from each other and the other members of FVAC.

In an emergency medical situation, bystanders can be part of the solution or they can be part of the problem. Calm and concerned friends or relatives can help to comfort and reassure a sick or injured patient. If they are hysterical, however, they can make a situation much worse by agitating a patient and interfering with rescuers. When I am crew chief, sometimes I have to decide quickly whether to allow a family member or dear friend to remain with a patient or not, depending on whether I believe he or she will make things better or worse. With children this can be a particularly difficult decision.

When I began in emergency work, I thought it would be wonderful to have a doctor or nurse stop at the scene to assist in caring for an injured victim. But I have found that although bystanders with medical training have the greatest potential for help, in an emergency situation they sometimes can be a hindrance.

* * *

As we approached the bad curve on Hunter's Hill Road, I could see the red glare of flares marking the scene of the accident. Sam Middleton, who was driving, slowed as we approached. We could see that a small Ford had tried to take the turn too fast and had skidded into a stone wall. The front end of the car was badly damaged and the windshield was shattered. A man was lying in the road next to the car. Fairfax Police Officer Chuck Harding directed us to pull over in front of the wreck and met me as I stepped out of the ambulance.

"What have you got, Chuck?" I asked him.

"One victim. She was alone in the car. A guy who seems to be a doctor stopped to help. He's with the patient now."

While my crew got the trauma kit and oxygen from the rig, I walked over to where a well-dressed, middle-aged man was kneeling over the body of an older woman. The man glanced up at me and I introduced myself. "Hi. My name's Ed Herman and I'm an EMT with the Fairfax Ambulance Corps."

"Get me some four-by-fours and a c-collar," he barked at me.

"My crew is bringing the crash kit with trauma dressings," I replied, moving to the patient's head and placing my hands firmly against her cheeks. "Try not to move your head," I said to her. "What's your name, ma'am?"

"Jane Seletsky," she replied. Jane had a large egg and a minor laceration on her forehead but otherwise her head and face did not appear to be injured. I looked at Jane's neck, then turned toward Sam and Fred Stevens, our third crew member, who were approaching with the trauma bag and oxygen. "We'll need a regular c-collar," I said.

Sam put down the oxygen and turned to go back to the ambulance for a regular-size cervical collar while Fred took over head stabilization so that I could examine Jane more thoroughly. "No," the man kneeling over the patient yelled. "I want a *tall*."

Sam turned toward me with a questioning look on his face. "Get both," I said. I was pretty sure that the correct size was regular, but it wouldn't hurt to bring a tall also. Turning toward my patient, I asked, "Where are you hurt?"

"Never mind that," the kneeling man barked. "She has head and facial lacerations. Everything else is okay. Just get a longboard and let's get her out of here."

"Excuse me, sir," I said through gritted teeth, "May I ask who you are?"

"I'm an army medic. The name's Andy Markbright."

Despite my growing irritation, I kept my voice calm. "Andy, I appreciate your help, but I am required to do my own patient survey." Sam had just returned with the two cervical collars. "Why don't you help Sam with putting on the c-collar," I suggested.

"You're doing what I already did," Andy muttered. "Damn waste of time."

I proceeded to question and examine Jane. "I understand that your head hurts. Do you hurt anywhere else?"

"I don't think so," the woman said hesitantly. "And everything moves okay."

I did a full patient survey and found that Andy had indeed been correct. Jane seemed to be uninjured except for her face and head. But facial and head injuries indicate the possibility of neck injury. Even though her neck appeared to be okay, we would have to do a full immobilization. I looked at the cervical collar that Andy had applied. It was a tall and it was forcing Jane's chin up, extending her neck into an awkward position. "Andy, would you please help Sam bring over a longboard, head blocks, and a spider strap?" I asked.

While Sam and Andy went to get the equipment, I quietly switched the tall collar for a regular while Fred continued to hold head stabilization. "Jane," I said, "we're going to immobilize you on a long backboard just as a precaution, to protect your neck and back while we transport you to the hospital. They'll check you out and fix the cuts on your head. Is that okay?"

"I guess," Jane said. "Am I really okay?"

"You're doing just great and we'll be out of here very quickly. Just be patient for a few more minutes."

"All right."

When Sam and Andy returned with the equipment, Sam placed the longboard on the ground next to Jane so that her legs extended beyond the bottom of the board. With the board in this position, we would be able to logroll her and pull her up onto the center of the board without needing to move her sideways. It was a trick not widely known by EMTs but one that we considered important as it avoids harmful movements of the patient's spine.

"The board's in the wrong place," Andy shouted, pushing the board down so that the bottom was flush with the victim's feet.

I took a deep breath and let it out slowly. "I want the board where Sam put it," I said, sliding the board up alongside Jane's body. "Watch how we do it. It works a lot better than the other way."

Andy grabbed the board and pulled it back down.

"This is where it belongs. You guys don't know what the fuck you're doing," he snapped.

I looked at the frightened expression on Jane's face, a common occurrence when rescuers argue about treatment in front of the patient. I had two choices. I could go along with Andy and continue to take orders from him, or I could do what I knew would minimize potential harm to the patient. I would not lose control of the situation. If I was going to do my job effectively, I couldn't allow that to happen.

I stood up. "Andy," I said, my voice soft but each word carefully enunciated, "can I talk to you?" I led him away from the patient. Then quietly but forcefully I continued, "Andy, I appreciate your assistance and I would like you to stay and help us. But I'm in charge and we're going to do it my way."

"Yeah," he hissed, "but you're fucking this all up."

"I don't care to hear your opinion," I said. "If you continue to interfere with me and my crew, I will have Officer Harding over there escort you from the scene, under arrest if necessary."

There was a second of dead silence while Andy took a deep breath. "Fuck you," he yelled, stomped to his car, and sped away, tires screeching.

Sam, Fred, and I completed our immobilization with no further problems and within ten minutes had Jane in the emergency room at FGH. She was treated and released the same day.

People with medical training can also be tremendously helpful.

I was in my car, on the way to get gas, when my pager began to beep. "GVK–861 Prescott headquarters to the

Rescue Squad. A full crew is needed to respond to a tractor-trailer versus bus PIAA at the intersection of Route 10 and Baxter."

I was on Route 10 just entering Prescott from Fairfax territory and Baxter was about a mile ahead. Since Prescott uses telephone to call in, I had no way to let them know I was responding so I switched on my blue light and drove toward the scene, thinking that I could ask someone at the scene to call headquarters for me.

A personal injury auto accident involving such large, heavy vehicles was potentially very serious, and I would probably be one of the first medical personnel at the scene. I felt a hollowness in the pit of my stomach. I don't like this at all, I thought, reviewing the priorities for a triage situation, one in which there are more victims than the available forces can handle.

About half a mile down the road, I heard a siren behind me. As I pulled over to let the fire engine pass I thanked God that Jack Johnson, the engine driver who was also an EMT, would get there before me.

As I rounded a bend in the road I saw the scene of the accident. The bus was in the middle of the intersection and the truck was a few hundred feet farther down the road. The truck had been carrying lumber, which was scattered like matchsticks over all four lanes. People were standing on the verge of the roadway, staring at the engine and the two crunched vehicles.

I pulled my car onto the shoulder, popped my trunk open, grabbed my crash kit, and trotted toward the bus, pulling on my gloves. The entire front end was crushed, and I could see that the driver was badly injured and trapped within the twisted metal. Jack was with him, holding his head while several more firefighters were setting up the Hurst Tool to cut away the metal that was pinning the driver. As he saw me approach, Jack leaned down and yelled through the bus's open front door. "The truck driver's okay, Ed. Check the bus passengers. You're on your own, since I'll need the medic here when he arrives."

"You got it, Jack."

I climbed into the bus and found a young woman kneeling next to an elderly man who was lying on his back in a pool of blood. His feet were under the driver's seat but fortunately were not entangled with the driver. Broken glass littered everything and the man's face was badly lacerated, with pieces of glass covering his skin. A teenage girl sat clutching her shoulder a few rows back, and in the seat behind her sat a young man, holding his left arm. The kneeling woman appeared to be uninjured.

"I'm an EMT with the Prescott Rescue Squad. My name is Ed," I said to her.

"I'm Diane," the young woman replied. "I'm an emergency room RN in the city."

I heaved a sigh, suddenly feeling not so alone and overwhelmed.

"I saw the accident happen," she continued. "This man"—she nodded toward the victim on the floor—"is the most seriously injured. We've got to get him out."

"What are his injuries?" I asked.

"Severe facial and head lacerations and swelling on both sides of his head. He's alert and oriented times three, his neuros are okay, and he doesn't seem to have any other injuries." With this first, complete, concise report, Diane immediately became part of my team.

"Have you checked out the other passengers?"

"Yes," Diane said. "The girl appears to have a shoulder

injury and the man is complaining only of wrist pain. I told them they'd have help in a minute, but they know that this guy's seriously injured. I think he should go first. Do you agree?"

I nodded, then leaned toward the fire chief who was helping with the driver. "Chief, are you sending the driver by ambulance?"

"No. We've got the helicopter on the way for him. The landing zone is in the shopping center so we can carry the driver to it on a longboard. I thought we could use the first rig to transport your patient."

"Good," I said. "Then all we'll need is a second rescue for the two walking wounded in the back."

"I'll take care of it, Ed," he said, pulling his radio from the pocket of his turnout coat. He would radio headquarters and update them as to our needs.

I returned my attention to Diane and my patient. "Did you get his vitals?"

"His pulse and respirations are within normal limits, but I don't have a BP cuff."

"Any LOC or SOB?"

"He denies loss of consciousness or shortness of breath."

Looking down at the man's position, I could see that we would have to move him as soon as we could. In addition to his injuries, his feet were interfering with the firefighters who were working to free the trapped driver.

"Diane, let's see whether we can slide him about five feet toward the back of the bus. Why don't you hold head stabilization and pull his shoulders while I keep his torso straight." I handed her a pair of gloves from among the several pairs I always have in my pockets and she pulled them on.

"Okay," Diane replied, placing her forearms on the sides of the man's head and her palms on his shoulders. Together we slid him back far enough to allow the extrication team room to maneuver.

With Diane holding head stabilization, I took out my BP cuff. "What's your name?" I asked the man.

"Chris," he replied softly.

"Chris, my name's Ed. I'm going to check your blood pressure and Diane will hold your head to keep it from moving. We'll get you out of here as quickly as we can." I heard the throb of the Hurst Tool start. "That's the cutting tool that is helping get the driver out," I yelled over the noise. "Just try to relax and we'll have you out of here in no time."

"I'll try," Chris replied.

Chris's blood pressure was normal. While we waited for the ambulance and more help to arrive, I removed a few pieces of glass from his face and dressed and bandaged his lacerations. Fortunately, none of the glass was embedded in his skin.

Although it seemed like hours, the ambulance arrived in only a few minutes. Several EMTs scrambled into the bus and began to care for the other two injured people. With Diane still holding his head and Prescott EMT Brenda Frost helping me, I applied a cervical collar to Chris's neck. Then we quickly slid our patient onto a longboard, strapped him down, and passed him out through the bus window to waiting firefighters. I wanted to kiss Diane for the great job that she had done but simply said, "Thanks a lot for your help," as I exited the bus to accompany my patient to the hospital.

I learned later that, once Chris was out of the bus, it took the rescue crew about fifteen more minutes to free the driver. By then a helicopter was waiting to transport him to St. Luke's Trauma Center. He was admitted in serious but stable condition and probably would be hospitalized for several more days. The girl with the injured shoulder and the man with pain in his wrist were transported to FGH by a second rescue vehicle, then treated and released. Chris was held overnight for observation, then released. The truck driver was uninjured.

Susan Whittier glanced out of the kitchen window. The school bus would come in about five minutes, so it was time to walk five-year-old Michael to the foot of the driveway, where the bus would pick him up. As usual, Michael had been ready for school early so she had let him play on the lawn. Suddenly Susan heard a shriek. She looked out and saw Michael lying on the ground. Dropping her jacket, Susan ran out to her son. "What happened?" she cried as she approached him.

"My neck, my neck," the little boy screamed.

"Michael, did you fall? Did something hit your neck?" she asked, trying to remain calm.

Michael continued shrieking. "No, no. But my neck hurts. I can't move it."

"Michael, don't move. I'm going to go into the house to call for help."

"Mommy, Mommy, don't go away," Michael screamed as Susan dashed into the house and dialed 911.

For most EMTs, saving a life and delivering a baby are two of the great highs of emergency medical work. Among volunteer EMTs, these experiences do not happen very often. But sometimes, unexpectedly,

I find that I get great satisfaction from much simpler accomplishments.

When Joan and I ride together, I usually let her take charge of rescue calls involving children. I feel helpless in dealing with shrieking, hysterical children whereas Joan seems to have a wonderful ability to calm them. But I was riding with an all-male crew when the call came in.

As we parked the ambulance in the driveway of the small two-story house on Poplar Street, I could see a little boy lying beside a low wall at the edge of a lawn. A young woman sat beside him and Police Officer Will McAndrews was kneeling, holding the boy's head. As I approached, the child began to scream and tried to pull Will's hands away from his head. "I don't wanna go in the ambulance," he screamed, kicking his heels against the wall.

"What happened?" I asked the woman, wondering how I was going to deal with the screaming boy.

"I don't know. He was playing on the lawn and he suddenly started screaming that his neck hurt."

"When did it happen?" I asked.

"About ten minutes ago."

"Has he been screaming like this since then?"

"Well, he started to calm down a little, but he started screaming again when he saw the ambulance."

"What's his name?"

"Michael."

It was obvious that we would need to immobilize Michael's neck and back in order to transport him to the hospital, but unless I could calm him, it was going to be a horrendous procedure. Clearly Michael was terrified. Forcibly tying him down, papoose style, would frighten him much more, and his struggles could worsen his neck injury. Furthermore, if he was so frightened by just seeing the ambulance, how would I ever be able to put an uncomfortable, hard cervical collar around his neck and completely immobilize him without scaring the shit out of him? But I had to try. I was crew chief and the other members of my crew were even more cowed than I was. The buck stopped with me.

I crouched, leaning toward the boy. His face was red, tear-streaked, and twisted with pain and fear. He was still trying to pull Will's hands away. "He's hurting my head," Michael shrieked. "Make him let go." Despite his mother's efforts to calm him he continued to squirm.

"Michael," I said softly yet firmly. "That's Officer McAndrews, and he's just holding your head still so that you don't hurt your neck any more. He wouldn't have to hold it so hard if you stop fighting with him."

Michael continued screaming and struggling.

"How old are you, Michael?" I asked.

"No, no," he shrieked. "Let me go."

"My name is Ed. I will be going in the ambulance with you," I said.

Michael screamed louder, his voice rising in pitch. "I don't wanna go in the ambulance. He's hurting me. You're gonna hurt me."

I placed my hands on both sides of Michael's head and nodded to Will to release his hold. Will sat back, relieved. "Michael," I said, "I'm holding your head now. But I won't have to hold it so tight if you don't try to move it. Okay?"

Michael tried to nod.

"Don't move your head when I ask you a question. Just say yes or no."

"Okay," Michael whimpered.

"Michael, I want to examine your neck. Okay?"

Michael shrieked. "No, no, you're gonna hurt me."

I continued clasping his head between my hands. "Michael," I said, looking directly into his eyes. "I want to tell you something. But you have to listen to me or you won't hear it."

Michael looked into my eyes and his cries diminished to a whimper.

"Michael," I said. "I never lie and I always keep my promises. And I promise you that I am not going to hurt you. Okay?"

"Are you sure?"

"I'm sure. And if I even make you blink, you can tell me to stop and I will. Are we agreed?"

"I guess," he whimpered.

"I'll just keep holding your head like I am. Can you show me where your neck hurts?"

Michael indicated a point to the right of his spinal column.

"Does it hurt when you touch it?" I asked.

"I don't know," he whimpered.

"Well, why don't you find out?"

Michael gingerly touched the spot and winced. "Yes," he replied.

"Does your neck hurt anywhere else?" I asked.

"No."

So far, so good, I thought. Michael had calmed down considerably. But how far would he let me go before becoming hysterical again?

By this time my crew members, Fred Stevens and Nick Abrams, had brought over the stretcher with a pediatric cervical collar, a pediatric immobilization board, and a stuffed bear. Fred came over and crouched next to me. "Do you like stuffed animals?" he asked Michael.

"Yes," Michael answered, no longer crying. Fred held out the stuffed bear with a plaid bow tie, which Michael snatched away and clasped to his chest.

"What do you say, Michael?" his mother said.

"Thank you."

"Michael, Fred is going to hold your head while I examine your neck. I'm going to touch you very gently, but if anything hurts when I touch it, you tell me and I'll stop right away."

"Okay," he said doubtfully.

Fred took over head stabilization and I gently touched Michael's toes. "Do these hurt?" I asked.

"No, it's my neck."

I tried to look very wise. "Oh. I was just making sure. Can you wiggle your toes for me?"

He did. I touched his hands. "Do these hurt?"

By this time Michael was looking at me as if I had lost my mind. "It's my neck, I said."

"Oh," I repeated. "Can you wiggle your fingers?" When he had moved his hands, I had him grasp my fingers in his and squeeze. The grip strength was equal and considerable. "Wow, you're strong." Then I palpated Michael's neck, avoiding the painful area. There was no need for me to determine exactly where the point tenderness was. Michael had done it for me. I quickly determined that there was no swelling, redness, deformity, or other areas of pain. It looked like Michael's injury was not serious and did not involve his spinal column. But we would have to do a complete immobilization anyway, just as a precaution.

I picked up the cervical collar and showed it to Michael.

"This is a collar that will protect your neck so that it won't hurt when we move you. I'm going to put it on you. May I do that?" I knew I was running a risk asking his permission, but if I gave him complete control and he let me immobilize his neck, our troubles were just about over.

"Okay," the boy said doubtfully.

I was home free. I quickly but gently applied the cervical collar, with no resistance from the child. "How does it feel?" I asked.

"I don't like it. It's hard and I can't move my head."

"I know it's uncomfortable, but moving your head will hurt your neck," I replied. "The collar will make sure that doesn't happen."

I held up the pediatric immobilization board and showed it to Michael. "We're going to put this behind you and slide you onto it. Then these flaps will cover you and keep you snug while we move you."

I demonstrated the Velcro immobilization flaps that would keep the child from moving. I hoped that Michael would experience the immobilization as being *snug* rather than *imprisoned*. It's amazing how the same physical experience can be so different depending on how you interpret it.

"I guess it'll be okay."

Michael whimpered a little as we completely immobilized him and carried him to the ambulance, but he did not resist. He chatted with me in the ambulance, telling me that his favorite TV shows were *Cops* and *Rescue 911*. When we arrived at FGH, Michael talked animatedly with the doctor and nurses. He was treated for a severe muscle spasm and released the same day.

It was a minor call, but it felt like a major accomplishment for me. I was quite certain that, because I succeeded in gaining the boy's trust, instead of remembering his EMS experience as one in which he was hurt, overwhelmed, and imprisoned despite his struggles, he would remember it as one in which he met some nice people who helped him and gave him a stuffed bear with a plaid bow tie.

Chapter 5

Over the years we have spent hundreds of hours in the emergency rooms of several area hospitals. We've brought hundreds of patients in via ambulance, we've volunteered, and we've observed. The only conclusion we've drawn is that nothing in an ER is ever predictable.

Thirteen-year-old Kathleen Shannahan was a redhead in every sense of the word. She had a face full of freckles, soft green eyes, and flaming red hair that wouldn't stay in any of the modern styles she tried out in the bathroom each weekend. In desperation she wore it in a fuzz around her face that looked like a cloud of red mist.

Kathleen also had the stereotypical redhead volatility, with a quick temper and an inability to sit still for long. She talked quickly, walked quickly, and had a tendency to inhale her food rather than eat it. A popular girl, her brief appearances at the dinner table each evening usually ended with the ringing of her phone and a dash up the stairs. Her own, separate phone number had been a thirteenth-birthday gift from her grandparents, but she worked around the house to earn enough to pay the basic monthly charges. Dutiful when she needed to be, she usually would gallop back down the stairs in time to stuff in a final mouthful of food and help her younger sister, Megan, put the last of the dishes into the dishwasher.

"Kathleen," her mother said as the phone rang one evening, "I will not have dinner interrupted one more time. Tell whoever it is that you cannot talk until at least 7:30, then come right back down here." As her daughter sprinted for the stairs, a roll in her hand, Mrs. Shannahan yelled, "If you aren't back here in sixty seconds I'll take the phone out, gift from your grand-mother or not." To her daughter's back, she finished, "Immediately."

In about five minutes, Kathleen reappeared. "Sorry, Mom."

"You bet you are, young lady," Mrs. Shannahan said. "New rule. No phone calls between 6:00 and 7:30. Period. And that goes for you too, Megan," she said, looking at Kathleen's ten-year-old sister, who only had an extension of her parents' phone in her room.

Kathleen plopped back into her seat and jammed a piece of roast beef into her mouth. "But, Mom," she said, barely chewing, "it's just this new science teacher. He's dumping gobs of work on us. Lab reports, homework, everything." She stuffed another piece of beef into her mouth and slugged a great swallow of Diet Pepsi. As she took a deep breath to continue her conversation, she felt the wad of half-chewed meat stick in her throat. She coughed and tried to take a breath but found she was unable to get any air past the lump. She coughed weakly, then, looking puzzled, stood up.

"Kathleen, sit down this instant," Mrs. Shannahan said, forking a French fry into her mouth and chewing delicately.

Kathleen's father, seated at the far end of the table, looked toward his elder daughter. "Kathleen, listen to your mother and sit down." He looked at her more closely, then said, "Are you all right?"

Silently Kathleen looked around the table, unable to understand why she couldn't catch her breath. From a distance she heard her father saying, "Kathleen Mary Shannahan, answer me." She could feel a great lump in her throat just at the hollow at the base of her neck.

Then everything happened at once. Mr. Shannahan, a technician at a local electronics assembly plant, stood up so quickly that his chair fell over backward. He came around behind his daughter, kicked her chair out of his way, and asked, "Are you okay? Can you talk to me?"

Kathleen tried to get a breath to answer but nothing moved. "It's okay," she heard her father say. "You've got something stuck in your throat. Right?"

She nodded, still disoriented. She felt her father reach around her and clasp his hands at her waist. "I know the Heimlich," he said calmly. "I can fix you right up. Try to stay calm."

Calm? How could she stay calm? She couldn't breathe. And how come he was so calm? Her hands shook and the trembling was rapidly taking over her entire body. She felt as if her father were punching her in her stomach. Over and over he jerked his clenched fists into her abdomen until suddenly she felt the piece of meat pop out of her mouth like the cork out of a champagne bottle. She gulped in a great breath of air.

"Darling." Her mother was at her side, hugging her. "Are you all right?"

She panted, alternately sucking in great lungfuls of air as quickly as she could and coughing, trying to relieve the tickle in her throat. Megan handed her a glass of water, and she sipped, trying to calm her shaking body. "I think"—she gasped—"I'm okay."

Megan used a napkin to pick up the half-chewed bite. "Gross," she muttered, wrapping a second napkin around the wad and heading for the kitchen. "Truly gross."

"Mike," Mrs. Shannahan said, "that was sensational. How did you know to do that?"

"The Heimlich maneuver was part of that CPR course I took when they made me area safety officer. Remember?"

"But that was years ago," Mrs. Shannahan said.

"Some things just stick with you, I guess," Mike Shannahan said, calmly sitting back down at the table and cutting another piece of beef.

Kathleen stood silently, trying to control the quakes that threatened to topple her. Slowly she sank into Megan's chair and put her head down on the table.

"Are you all right now, honey?" her mother asked.

"I'm okay." She panted, grateful for every mouthful of air she could get, rubbing the sore spot where the lump had been. Eventually the pain dissipated and her breathing slowed.

"Oh, baby," her mother said, picking up her chair and pulling it up beside her. "I have never been so frightened." She enveloped her daughter in a great bear hug. "Don't ever do that to me again."

"Dad," Megan said, returning from the kitchen, "you were awesome."

Slowly the family returned to normal. By the following morning, except for Kathleen's feelings of gratitude to her father, the incident was all but forgotten.

The next day was unusually quiet at Kathleen's school.

She had an entire day with no tests, she wasn't called on in Spanish, and Bobby Camarillo actually said hi to her as they passed in the hall between fourth and fifth period. As she sat on the bus, she began to have a pain in her chest, under the upper end of her breastbone, right below the hollow at the base of her neck. Just that lump from last night, she thought. No sweat.

As the bus made its many stops before Kathleen's, she began to worry about the pain. Remembering what her health teacher had said about heart attacks and chest pain, she started to become concerned. That big bone down the center of her chest—the sternum, Mrs. Haverstraw had called it. Substernal chest pain is a sure sign of a heart attack. I'm having a heart attack, Kathleen decided. She felt her body tremble and sweat prickle under her arms. Her heart pounded and her breathing quickened.

By the time she reached her bus stop, she was convinced that she was dying. She staggered into the house and yelled for her mother. A school monitor, her mother usually got home before her. "Mom," she shrieked. "Help."

Mrs. Shannahan rocketed from the kitchen. "What's the matter, baby?"

"I think I'm dying." She panted. "Chest pain."

"Get into the car," Mrs. Shannahan snapped. "Now!"

With Kathleen gasping for breath in the passenger seat, Mrs. Shannahan drove to the trauma center and double-parked in front of the emergency entrance. "Hurry inside," she said, trying to get the keys out of the ignition while the car was still in drive.

As Kathleen got out of the car, a man in navy pants and a white uniform shirt with a security patch on the sleeve hustled to the driver's side window. "Ma'am," he said, "you can't leave this here."

"But my daughter's dying."

The guard looked at the teenager, whose face was flushed and breathing was rapid, and said, "I'll help her inside. You can put your car right there." He pointed to a parking space with the words ER ONLY painted on the pavement in front of it.

"But she needs me."

"I'll take care of her," the guard said, walking over to Kathleen and draping his arm around her shoulders. "You put the car away."

As her mother restarted the car, the guard said to Kathleen, "Can you stand there a moment while I get you a wheelchair?"

She bent over, placed her hands on her thighs, and, barely able to breathe, nodded. The guard left and, a moment later, returned and guided her into a wheelchair. Inside, they stopped at the triage desk where Kathleen, between gulping breaths, gave her name and address to the woman behind the desk. The receptionist picked up a phone, dialed a number, and, over the loudspeaker, Kathleen heard, "A nurse to the triage desk, please."

Mrs. Shannahan ran up to the desk just as a woman in purple scrubs arrived from behind a swinging door. The scrub-clad woman spoke quickly to the triage nurse, then hurried to Kathleen. "Hello, Kathleen. I'm Erika Morely. Tell me what you're feeling right now."

"Hard to get my breath," Kathleen said. "Pain in my chest."

"Point to where it hurts," Erika said, and Kathleen pointed to the upper end of her sternum with her index finger. "Is it a sharp pain or a dull one?"

"Sharp."

"Does it travel to anywhere else? Your back, or belly or arm or neck?"

"Not really," Kathleen said, still panting.

"What do you think is wrong, Doctor?" Mrs. Shannahan asked.

"I'm a nurse," Erika said, "and we don't have enough information yet." She turned to Kathleen. "Do you have any other symptoms? Anything at all?"

"My arms feel funny."

"How funny?"

"Numb sort of. And my lips too. And my hands feel funny too."

She saw that the girl's color was good, no blue tinge around her lips, and took in all the other symptoms. A small smile appeared on Erika's face. "Well, Kathleen," she said, picking up a handful of papers, "I think you're just breathing too fast. Try to slow your breathing down as best you can and don't breathe as deeply as you are. Can you try that while we take you inside?"

"I guess," Kathleen replied, making a conscious effort to slow her breathing the way the nurse said.

"That's good. Let's take you back into the emergency room and check you out, but I think this isn't serious at all."

"Really?" Kathleen and her mother said together.

Erika squeezed the girl's shoulder and nodded.

"Can I come with her?" Mrs. Shannahan asked.

"You're her mother?"

"Yes."

"You can meet us in a moment. Just give the triage nurse your insurance information, sign some forms, then follow us through that door. You'll find us in one of the cubicles. I'll leave word." She pushed the wheelchair through the set of swinging doors through which she had arrived.

Kathleen was overwhelmed by the confusion of sights, smells, and sounds. A dozen scrub-clad people bustled efficiently from place to place. Three people in white lab coats stood behind a massive counter, talking on phones. The area smelled like the bathroom after her mother cleaned it, and several conversations were going on at once. "Wow," Kathleen said.

"It's quite busy this afternoon," Erika said as she wheeled Kathleen into a curtained cubicle. She handed the girl a white garment with faded blue dots. "I need you to take off your clothes, everything but your panties, and put this on with the opening in the back."

Kathleen continued to breathe rapidly. "Slow that breathing down," Erika said. "I'm going to get something for you to breathe into."

Erika Morely was pretty sure that Kathleen was hyperventilating as she presented all the information to Maria Sanchez, the pediatric attending physician that afternoon. When she had finished, Dr. Sanchez said, "Sounds like you're right, Erika, but let's do an EKG, check her PO_2, and do some blood work just to be sure. And we need a paper bag. Where do we keep them?" Having Kathleen breathe into a paper bag would reduce the amount of oxygen in each inhalation and, the doctor hoped, break the cycle of hyperventilations.

"I haven't a clue." More loudly, the nurse said, "Anyone know if we have any paper bags?" When several of the nurses looked blank, Erika continued, "Okay, anyone have a bag lunch?"

A nurse appeared from a trauma room. "I don't have a lunch," she said, "but I have some crackers in my purse."

Several of the people around the desk laughed. "We need the bag, not the lunch," Erika said. "We've got a kid hyperventilating."

"Oh," the nurse said, "sorry. I guess breathing in the cracker package won't do."

Several more people laughed. "How about a non-rebreather mask?" Carol Marks, an EMT and ER nurse, asked. "If you pull off the flaps covering the outlet ports and don't connect it to the oxygen, it might do that same thing."

"Hey, Carol, great idea," Erika said, getting the required mask. "Where did you get that one?"

"Someone mentioned it in my last EMT refresher course."

Erika grabbed a non-rebreather oxygen mask from the basket, pulled the rubber covers from the side ports of the mask, and walked back into Kathleen's cubicle. She clipped the finger element of the pulse oximeter onto the girl's index finger. "This will show us how your blood's doing." The reading was 98, showing that her blood was richly oxygenated and all but confirming her diagnosis. "That's very good, Kathleen. You're blood's in terrific shape." She handed the mask to the flushed girl. "Here, breathe into this. Hold it against your face and breathe slowly."

Then she wheeled a large machine into the cubicle. "This machine will tell us about how your heart's beating." She placed sticky tabs down the center of the girl's chest, across her ribs, one on each arm, and one on each thigh. "I need you to try to relax and sit very still so I can get a good look." For several minutes Erika watched the spiky line travel across the screen. "Looks fine to me." She checked the girl's vital signs and wrote them on her chart. "Tell me about school. What grade are you in?"

Dr. Sanchez walked into the cubicle, interrupting the conversation. "How do you do, Kathleen. I'm Dr. Sanchez, the attending pediatrician this afternoon. How are you feeling?"

As Kathleen explained, Dr. Sanchez studied the line on the screen, then printed a strip on paper. "Well, your EKG is normal." She looked at the vitals Erika had written. "All these are within normal limits. Your heartbeat's a bit fast and we know your breathing's fast too. Everything points to a sort of panic attack. The chest pain puzzles me, however. Have you had any illness like bronchitis, a heavy cough, anything like that in the last week or so?"

Kathleen looked at her mother and put the mask aside. Together the two women said, "The meat."

"Meat?"

They told Dr. Sanchez about the choking incident from the previous evening. "I had almost forgotten about it," Mrs. Shannahan said. "It all happened so fast."

Dr. Sanchez grinned at Kathleen. "I'll bet it didn't seem fast to you."

Through the mask, Kathleen replied, "Not at all. It felt like about a week. I remembered it on the bus, but then I just sort of forgot."

"How are your hands and lips?"

"Better," Kathleen said, her breathing slowing.

"Well, we're going to do a few more tests and let you stay for a little while until you feel normal again, but I think you're just fine."

Three hours later, with a clean bill of health, Kathleen and her mother left the trauma center. "Well, my love," Mrs. Shannahan said, starting the car, "the dinner I had planned is history. What would you like?"

"Anything but roast beef."

"Yeah," Mrs. Shannahan said, "good thinking."

Tie still untied, jacket over his arm, Brad Garvey dashed out of the house and slammed the front door behind him. Late for work as usual, he yanked his car door open and climbed behind the wheel. He stabbed the key into the ignition and turned. Nothing. No grind. No grunt. Not even a click. Nothing. He reached for the headlight switch and found it in the "on" position. "Shit," he muttered. "Shit, shit, shit."

He ran back to the front door, pulled it open, and yelled, "Honey, I'm taking your car. Mine's dead. Ask one of your friends to come over and jump it, then take my car for the day. I'll call you later." Without waiting for an answer, he dashed for his wife's Toyota, climbed behind the wheel, and turned the key in the ignition. It started immediately. "Thank God," he said. He knew that the Toyota had been having overheating problems and was annoyed that his wife had delayed the trip to the mechanic. As he drove toward the parkway, he watched the temperature gauge but, although it was higher than it should have been, it stayed well outside of the red zone.

Brad waited impatiently for a break in the parkway traffic. "Damn," he spat as a Lexus sped by him. "Can't the bastards let anyone in?" He tromped on the gas and slipped into the stream of city-bound traffic. Brad saw his wife's water bottle on the seat beside him and lifted it to his mouth. Thirsty after his previous excitement, he took a long drink. The water tasted funny, almost sweet, and he stared at the container. "What has that woman been drinking?" It took only a few seconds for him to make the connection. "That was antifreeze," he yelled. "Shit. I've been poisoned."

Weaving through traffic, he pulled his cell phone from his pocket and dialed 911.

"County 911. What is your emergency?"

"I think I just drank antifreeze. Is it poisonous?"

"I'm afraid I don't know that, sir. You're on a cell phone?"

"Yes."

"If you'll tell me your location, I'll have an ambulance and a paramedic pick you up."

"Never mind that," Brad said, and pushed the DISCONNECT button. Steering with one hand, he dialed his doctor's number with the other. When the nurse answered he said without preamble, "Is antifreeze poisonous?" He slammed the brake as a station wagon braked in front of him.

"Who is this?" the nurse asked.

"Just ask Dr. McClarron if antifreeze is poisonous. Please."

As static filled the air, Brad's palms began to sweat and he felt lightheaded. He had no idea whether it was from the stress or the poison. He considered pulling over, then decided to get closer to the next exit.

He heard the sounds of the phone being picked up. "Antifreeze can be deadly," Dr. McClarron said into the phone. "Who is this?"

"It's Brad Garvey," Brad said. "What should I do?"

"Call 911 and get to the emergency room. It can be treated easily, but you need to do that quickly."

As Brad pushed the DISCONNECT button he saw the large blue and white "H" on the sign at the Oakmont exit. He turned off and headed for the hospital's emergency room. Now his heart was pounding and his breathing was rapid. He followed the signs for St. Luke's Trauma Center, swerved into a parking space behind the ER, and rushed in the door. "I've been poisoned," he said to the triage nurse who took his information and got a quick reading on his vital signs.

"Nurse to triage," she then said into the loudspeaker.

Someone in light-green scrubs hustled him through the doors and into a cubicle. A tall slender woman with a black braid that hung halfway down her back arrived soon thereafter. "I'm Dr. Janine Singh and I'm the attending physician this morning. Tell me what happened."

"I've told seventy-eight people already. I drank antifreeze."

Familiar with drunks who occasionally drank antifreeze, knowing only that it was alcohol, Dr. Singh was amazed that this well-dressed business type had deliberately consumed the chemical. "How did you happen to do that?"

"My wife's been having car trouble, the radiator's been losing water. I guess she filled a water bottle with water and antifreeze and when I took her car this morning, I accidentally drank some." He was feeling awful, shaky, sweaty, and terrified.

"Okay, Mr. Garvey, just try to relax. I know you're frightened, but be assured that we can fix this problem. You're going to be just fine."

Brad took a deep breath and tried to calm his racing heart. "Are you sure?"

Dr. Singh perched on the edge of the bed and took

Brad's wrist to again check his pulse. "Do you know about how much you drank?"

"I don't know how much was water and how much was antifreeze in the bottle. But it tasted very sweet."

"How long ago?"

"Maybe twenty minutes. Are you going to have to pump my stomach or make me throw up?"

"I don't think so since a lot of the chemical is already in your bloodstream. What we are going to do is give you an antidote, and it's going to be really strange."

Brad raised an eyebrow. "Strange?"

"Yes. The antidote is liquor."

Brad's eyes widened. "Booze?"

Dr. Singh grinned. "Yup. To make it a little easier to understand, what we have to do is overwhelm the bad alcohol, that's the methyl alcohol in the antifreeze, with good alcohol, that's ethyl alcohol like scotch or vodka. We may have it in a form we can give you as an IV, or we may have to get you drunk."

"You're kidding."

Dr. Singh raised an eyebrow and just smiled.

"Awesome," Brad said. "You mean I'll have to miss work? Doctor's orders?"

"I'm afraid so. You can call or we can if you like."

"Miss a day of work and get drunk. Hmmm. You know, Doc, I think I love you."

Dr. Singh returned about fifteen minutes later with her hand behind her back. "I called the hospital pharmacy and unfortunately we have no IV ethyl alcohol. One of the nurses lives nearby and got this for you." She pulled a bottle of vodka from behind her back and Brad grinned. "Orange juice with it all right with you?"

"Sure." Finally realizing that this was all serious, Brad

pulled off his jacket and tie, kicked off his shoes, and put his feet up on the stretcher. Five minutes later he was holding a paper cup filled to the brim with orange liquid, heavy on the vodka.

"Drink this down rather quickly, then pour yourself another." Dr. Singh looked at her watch. "It's almost nine thirty. I'd like you to have three of these before noon."

"You're on, Doc." He raised the cup in a mock salute, then downed half the cupful in one long gulp.

Two hours later, Dr. Singh ushered Brad's wife into the cubicle. "Brad," Ruth Garvey said, "you're really all right. That was such a stupid thing I did, leaving that water bottle there yesterday. I had no idea you'd be taking my car."

"It's fine, Ruth," Brad said, now well into his third screwdriver. "No sweat." He turned to the doctor, who had completed another set of vitals. "How am I doing?" He knew that his speech was a bit slurred, but he was floating so lightly that he didn't care.

"You're just great. We'll keep you around for a few more hours and do some more blood tests, just to be sure, but by midafternoon you'll be out of here."

"Listen, Doc, can you get some sand brought in?" He winked at the two women. "Ruthie and I have always wanted to go to Club Med." He pulled his wife's arm until she was sitting on the stretcher beside him. Then he kissed her noisily. "Haven't we?"

Ruth just giggled.

Ten-year-old Damian Jefferson had gone to his best friend Juan Ramirez's house after school one Wednesday afternoon. Although it was March, there was no sign of spring in the air and, as a cold rain fell, the boys pined for the warmer weather. "God, I hate this cold," Damian said as they lay on old mattresses in Juan's basement.

"We could go up to my room," Juan said, his brown eyes appearing deeply concerned. "We could play Nintendo."

"Nah," Damian said. "This is the place, man." He inhaled the slightly musty smell and watched dust motes dance in the late-afternoon light. He spread his arms and banged more dust from the wide mattress on which the two boys sprawled. "Your folks are the greatest. Lettin' you use this room and all."

Juan grinned. "You wouldn't say that if you had to sit through church with them every Sunday."

"Yeah, that's a bummer," Damian said. "It was great before they made you go with them." Damian knew that two months ago, on Juan's tenth birthday, the Ramirezes had announced that Juan was now old enough to go with them regularly and "sit and behave" as Juan frequently mimicked. The boys used to enjoy Sunday mornings at Damian's house when the Ramirezes used to drop Juan off and pick him up several hours later.

"Got any homework?" Juan asked, deliberately changing the subject.

"Yeah. I got math problems and a thing for Ms. Waterman on the French and Indian War." He made a rude noise. The boys weren't in the same class in school this year, and not being able to share assignments made homework all the more painful. "You?"

"Math too, but we're still on the Revolution. Gotta read four pages on Patrick Henry."

"Bummer," Damian said. Then he sat up. "Did your dad ever get that new fishing stuff?"

"Hey, yeah. Lemme get it and show you." He galloped upstairs and returned with several brown-paper packages, which he slowly unwrapped. "First day of the season and we're off."

"Lucky," Damian said.

Juan looked at his best friend and slowly a grin lit up his face. "I got a surprise for you." Damian held his breath and crossed his fingers as Juan continued. "You can come along if your folks let you. I asked my dad and he said yes."

Damian felt his heart pound. "He did?" He had been afraid to ask Juan to ask his dad, but Juan had anyway. He was a real friend. "That's fan-fuckin'-tastic."

"Do you think your folks will let you?"

"Yeah, I guess. Sure. Why not?"

The two boys high-fived each other, then Juan laid out the now-unwrapped equipment on the mattress between them. He got a green metal box from the corner of the basement and opened it reverently. "Lemme show you this stuff." For the next half hour, Juan gave Damian a guided tour of the new purchases and his father's tackle box, explaining different types of lures. Then he got his father's fly rod from the corner and fastened a particularly interesting-looking green plastic blob with three hooks to the end of the line. "It's got a fancy name, but my dad calls it Hector."

"Hector?"

"He said that the guy who first taught him to use this was named Hector so . . ." Juan stood up and began to flick the end of the rod. "My dad says that you have to caress the water surface like a woman." He giggled and blushed a bit, and soon the two boys were laughing, holding their stomachs.

As he pulled himself together, Juan again began to flick the tip of the rod. "Can you make that thing work?" Damian asked.

"My dad can land this thing in a circle two feet around from fifty feet away." Juan rummaged behind an old dresser and finally came out with an old hula hoop. "You gotta practice until you can cast the lure into the water just over old Mr. Fish's head." He handed the rod to Damian, crossed the basement, and put the hoop on the ground. He returned and took the rod back. "Like this," he said. He flicked the tip of the rod and the lure landed on the dresser at the far end of the basement.

Damian giggled. "Not like that, man," he said.

Juan laughed. "Well, not exactly. But it's really hard."

"Lemme try."

The two boys took turns trying to land the green plastic lure with the three barbed hooks attached inside the hula hoop. On Juan's turn, he flicked the rod and suddenly Damian screamed. "What happened?" Juan yelled, then realized that the lure had lodged itself behind Damian's right ear. "Sorry, man," he said, pulling the line. "Is it tangled in your hair?"

"No, you asshole," Damian said as he grabbed the fishing line and yanked, pulling the rod from Juan's hand. Then he sat down on the floor with a thud. "It's in my ear!"

Juan ran to his friend's side, pulled Damian's earlobe away from the green plastic, and peered behind. "Man, it's really hooked in there," he said.

"I know that, you idiot. Get it out!"

Juan grabbed the lure and tried to pull the hook out. "Ow," Damian yelled. "Let me do that." He felt around, grasped the plastic part, and moved it around every which way.

"Does it hurt, man?" Juan said, crouching and staring at Damian's ear, his eyes wide. "It's really stuck in your skin."

"It doesn't tickle." Damian wiggled the lure, but any way he moved it, it hurt more. "Oh, shit. I can't get the damn thing out. Is it bleeding?"

"No, it's not bleeding but it's caught by the barbs, those little hook things. It won't come out."

"Well, get it out."

Again Juan tried to push and pull the hook but it was stuck fast. When it began to make his ear hurt more, Damian said, "Hey, that really hurts. Stop! Stop it!"

Juan got a pair of scissors and cut the fishing line, then sat back on his haunches and said, "So now what? My folks aren't home so I guess we have to call your mom. You can't leave that thing in there."

"Oh, swell," Damian muttered, knowing the hell he'd catch. Realizing he had no other real choice, he phoned his mother at work, glad that it was almost five and she'd be getting off anyway.

"You did *what*?" Mrs. Jefferson said into the phone from her seat at the main phone at the local Buick dealer.

The pain was almost gone but Damian knew how to handle his mother. "I'm sorry, Mom, but it really hurts. It's caught in my ear. In the back. We can't get it out."

"Are you okay? Does it hurt bad?"

Mrs. Jefferson's voice was loud so Juan could hear both ends of the conversation. "It was bleeding before, but it stopped," Damian said, rolling his eyes. He covered the mouthpiece so his mother wouldn't hear Juan giggling. When the noise subsided, he lifted his hand and said, "It really hurts."

Damian could hear his mother's deep breath. "Okay, baby," she said. "I was getting ready to leave so I'm ready. I'll pick you up there in fifteen minutes. Try to be brave." She hung up.

"It was bleeding but I'll try to hang on," Juan mimicked as Damian hung up the phone. "You're so full of shit."

Damian giggled. "Well, if she learns that this is really so lame and that I'm not really hurt, just stuck, I'll really catch hell. And I do have to get this fucker out of there."

When Mrs. Jefferson arrived, she peered at the lure, then wiggled the hooks. "Oh, baby," she said. "I can't get it out."

Tears of frustration and embarrassment were just beneath the surface but Damian blinked them back. "So what do we do now?"

Half an hour later, Damian lay on a gurney in the emergency room at St. Luke's. A woman with dark-brown skin, deep brown eyes, and a heavy Spanish accent walked through the door toward Damian and his mother. She was tiny with short, straight hair, a stethoscope around her neck, and a white lab coat covering her jeans and bright red polo shirt. She looked not too much older than Juan's seventeen-year-old sister.

"Hello there," the woman said, looking at the handful of papers she carried. "You must be Damian Jefferson. I'm Dr. Sanchez." She looked Damian directly in the eye and put out her hand. Damian shook it.

"Are you a real doctor?"

"Don't be rude, young man," Mrs. Jefferson said.

"That's all right, ma'am," Dr. Sanchez said. She looked at Damian. "Yes, I'm a real doctor."

"You look like my friend's sister."

The doctor grinned. "I know I look really young, but I assure you I've been through medical school and internship and I've been working here for three years."

"Oh," Damian said.

"Now, Damian," Dr. Sanchez said, "why don't you tell me what happened?" She rounded the stretcher so she could look at the lure with its fishhook embedded behind the boy's ear.

"He and his friend were playing and he got that thing caught," Mrs. Jefferson said.

"I'm sure he did," Dr. Sanchez said, "but I would like to hear Damian tell me about it."

Damian grinned. It wasn't often that someone wanted to talk to him and not to his mother. "My friend Juan was showing me how to cast and this thing got caught in my ear."

"You didn't fall or anything when this happened?"

"No."

"Well then, there's one other important question," Dr. Sanchez said, then paused.

"What's the problem?" Mrs. Jefferson asked, her brow suddenly wrinkling. "He's had all his shots."

Dr. Sanchez winked, then leaned over and spoke into Damian's ear. "The question is"—she paused for effect, then continued—"now that you're hooked and reeled in, should we keep you or throw you back?"

Damian grinned for the first time since the family had arrived at the hospital. "Keep me," he said softly.

"Well, all right then," Dr. Sanchez said. "I guess

we have to get this thing out from behind your ear, don't we?"

Damian's heart began to pound. "I guess." This whole ridiculous thing was getting more and more complicated, and his ear was really getting sore.

"We'll do it easily and it will hardly hurt. I promise, and I never lie to my patients." Somehow, Damian believed her.

"You said that he's had all his school shots?" the doctor asked.

"Of course," Mrs. Jefferson answered.

"I don't think the hook is in the cartilage so it shouldn't be too hard to get it out. I'll be right back with more tools. You know, Damian, we have all sorts of instruments and things to help injured people. But to help you, I need some wire cutters and a pair of pliers from the maintenance department."

"Is he going to be okay?" Mrs. Jefferson asked.

"Of course. Don't you worry." She turned her attention to the boy. "I'm going to take your blood pressure, Damian. You've had that done before, right?"

Damian nodded.

Dr. Sanchez wrapped a BP cuff around the boy's upper arm. She pumped it up, then, with her stethoscope on the inside of his elbow, watched the gauge as the squeezing released. Then she held his wrist and gazed off into space. She looked into his eyes and stuck a plastic thing into his good ear. "This is a fancy thermometer so I can take your temperature." The machine beeped. "Your temperature is normal, and your blood pressure, pulse, and breathing are just fine. I'll see what we can get from maintenance and I'll be back in a few minutes."

"Okay," Damian said. He looked at his mom. She had

been surprisingly tolerant about this mess, and now he wondered whether he could push his luck. "Mom," he said, trying to look pained. "I'm kinda hungry."

"Well," Mrs. Jefferson said, patting Damian on his shoulder, "what can we do about that?"

He tried to look as if he were in great pain but hiding it. "I saw a candy machine on the way in here," he said, knowing his mother's feelings about sugar.

He watched as his mother fumbled in her purse and found her wallet. "I suppose this time. Just this once."

Softly, looking injured, Damian whispered, "Snickers?"

"You're being so brave. I think we can manage that."

Some time later, Dr. Sanchez returned. "Okay, I've got some wire cutters and a pair of pliers that I think will do the trick." She showed the pliers to Damian and said, "This might hurt a bit. I can give you a shot to numb the area, or we can try without. Your choice."

My choice, Damian thought. Dynamite. Much as the ear was now sore as hell and he'd love a shot, he was a man. "Just go ahead," he said, rolling onto his left side.

"Okay," the doctor said. "Here's what we're going to do." As she explained, the doctor ministered to Damian's ear from behind him. "First a little alcohol, both on the pliers and on your ear. It might sting a little."

A little? Damian thought. It felt like a hot poker was thrust through the back of his ear. This hurt more than anything that had happened all day.

"Okay, now I'm going to cut the back end of this." There was a loud snapping sound. "And this end too." Another snip. Then the body of the green plastic lure landed on the stretcher beside him and he heard a *clink* as what must have been the other end was deposited in the garbage can. "This part might hurt a bit too," the doctor said.

"Ow," Damian said despite his personal vow not to make a sound.

"Sorry, Damian," the doctor said. Another *clink* and the final piece of the lure landed in the garbage can.

"Yeah," Damian answered, surprised as the pain subsided as quickly as it had started. "No biggie."

"Okay, we're done," Dr. Sanchez said. She rubbed some smelly stuff over the area then spread goop over it. "Keep it clean and dry for twenty-four hours," she continued, "then forget it."

"Thank you so much, Doctor," Mrs. Jefferson said.

"Yeah," Damian said as he sat up. "Thanks, Doc."

"That's *doctor*," Mrs. Jefferson corrected him.

"Doc is fine and you were great," Dr. Sanchez said. "And no more fooling around with fishing lures. I don't want to see you here again."

Damian sat up, his head aching a bit but otherwise none the worse for the experience. "Yeah, Doc, me too. I'm out of here?"

"You're gone," the doctor said, picking up her tools. "Mrs. Jefferson, he was great. You've got a wonderful boy here."

"Well, thank you," Mrs. Jefferson said.

As he watched Dr. Sanchez leave, Damian said, "You know, Mom, we have to pass that candy machine on the way out too."

"I didn't know what else to do, Doctor," Amanda Cross said to the calm, white-coated woman who entered the trauma cubicle. With her left hand she pulled a handkerchief from her purse and dabbed at her nose. Her right hand never left the grasp of the four-year-old girl on the stretcher.

"Calm down," Dr. Sanchez said, quickly reading the chart the nurse handed her. She looked at the little girl, whose head was filled with tiny braids, each tipped with a colored barrette. The girl had a white towel wrapped around her right forearm. "Hi, Viola," she said softly to the girl. "I'm Dr. Sanchez."

Silently the girl turned her head toward her mother, away from the doctor.

"What happened, Mrs. Cross?" Dr. Sanchez asked, gently taking the girl's arm and checking the pulse below the injury.

"She was playing in the backyard. We have a fence and I just didn't expect anything. She was just playing." She dabbed at her nose again.

"How long ago did this happen?"

Mrs. Cross looked at her watch. "About three hours ago."

"Okay, and how did she hurt herself?"

"She told me a cat scratched her. The scratches were pretty deep and I thought she might need stitches."

Dr. Sanchez gently and slowly unwrapped the towel with her gloved fingers. She saw that the inner layers were bloody but not blood-soaked.

"Ow," the little girl said. "Hurts."

"She's a very tough girl," Dr. Sanchez said to Mrs. Cross. "She's not crying. Did she cry when this happened?"

"Not too much," Mrs. Cross said. "She was just mad that the cat ran away."

Dr. Sanchez's attention returned to the girl. "Viola, I'm sorry I hurt you. Does it hurt very much?"

The little girl stared at the doctor, stuck out her lower lip, and nodded.

"Your mommy says a kitty scratched you." She examined the three, closely spaced, deep grooves in the tiny deep-brown forearm. "Was it your kitty?"

"We don't have animals," Mrs. Cross said.

"I want Viola to tell me," Dr. Sanchez said. "Viola? Do you know that kitty?"

When the girl hesitated, her mother said, "Tell the doctor, Viola."

When the girl remained silent, Dr. Sanchez asked, "Was it a white kitty?"

The girl shook her head, and her barrettes clicked against each other.

"Well," Dr. Sanchez said, using a tweezers to pull white threads from the towel away from the ripped skin, "that's very interesting. Was it brown?"

Again the head shook.

"I'll bet I know," Dr. Sanchez said. "I'll bet it was green." When the girl's head shook wildly, Dr. Sanchez continued. "Yes. That's right. Green with red stripes."

"No, it wasn't."

Dr. Sanchez tried to look surprised. "It wasn't?"

"No, silly."

"Maybe blue and purple."

"No. It was gray."

"Oh," Dr. Sanchez said. "It was gray. No stripes?"

"It had stripes on its tail," Viola said.

Now suspicious, Dr. Sanchez said, "I'm going to wash this arm while you tell me more about the kitty. It might hurt a little. Is that okay?"

"Do you have to?"

"I'm afraid I do. I wish I could do it without hurting

you, but it should only hurt a little." She nodded at Erika Morely, the nurse who had accompanied her into the cubicle, and Erika opened a bottle of sterile water and unwrapped several 4 × 4 dressings.

"Okay," Viola's tiny voice said.

"Tell me about this kitty. You said it was blue, with a yellow-striped tail."

"No." Viola giggled. "It was gray with black stripes on his tail."

As she gently washed the girl's arm, she continued, "And I'll bet it had a silly mask on its face over his eyes."

"How did you know?" the girl asked.

"I just guessed." She looked up at Mrs. Cross. "I suspect that she found a small raccoon."

"Oh, God," Mrs. Cross cried. "A raccoon. They carry rabies. She's going to die."

Tears welled in Viola's eyes and trickled down her cheeks.

"Of course not." Glaring at the woman, furious at her for frightening the girl, Dr. Sanchez stroked the small forehead with her forearm. "It's okay, baby," she said. "There's nothing to be afraid of at all. I promise."

"That's right darling. Mommy's sorry. Everything's going to be fine. Really." She turned to the doctor. "We'll talk later," she said conspiratorially.

"We can talk now. I have no secrets from my patient." She grinned at Viola. "That's you."

A small smile replaced her tears but her lower lip quivered.

"Viola, listen to me." Dr. Sanchez continued to clean the clotted blood from the deep, ugly scratches on the girl's arm. "I swear that I'll tell you everything. Okay?"

After a moment's deep consideration, the girl said, "Okay."

"Now here's what's going to happen. First I'm going to finish cleaning these nasty scratches. Do they hurt a lot?"

"Not too much."

"That's great, honey. After I get you cleaned up, I'm going to have to take a few stitches so your arm will heal cleanly and stay beautiful." She glared at Mrs. Cross, who remained silent.

"Stitches?"

"Yes. But I'll give you some medicine so it won't hurt at all."

"Needles?"

"Yes. The medicine I give you will be in a needle, but you'll only feel a little stick. Then I'll fix up your arm just fine. You'll have to come back and visit me a few times after that."

"Why?"

"Well," Dr. Sanchez said, finishing the careful washing of the injury by scrubbing the entire area with Betadyne, "I'll have to take out the stitches, which will pinch a little but not much more. And also, Mommy is going to have to call the health department to get some special medicine for you."

"Why?"

"I think you were scratched by a raccoon and he might have been sick. We need to give you medicine so you won't get sick too."

"But he wasn't sick."

"Yes, I'm afraid he was. Raccoons like to come out at night. They're very scaredy animals and they don't much like people."

"He liked me."

"I think he liked you because he wasn't feeling too well. You know how you like to be cuddled when you don't feel well? I think your raccoon wanted that too."

"Oh." Viola's eyes didn't leave Dr. Sanchez's hands as the doctor gathered the stitching paraphernalia.

"You've never seen that animal before, have you?"

"No."

"Or anyone like him?"

"No."

"It's important that you don't touch any animal that you don't know. Will you promise me?"

"Okay."

"I think Mommy should tell the police about your animal so someone can try to catch him."

"What will they do to him?"

"I don't know. But if he's sick they need to keep him from biting or scratching some other little girl like you. You don't want someone else to get hurt, do you?"

"I guess not."

Erika handed Dr. Sanchez the numbing agent. "I'm going to put some medicine into your arm that will make it not feel anything later. It will stick a little but that's all. Are you ready?"

"I guess."

"Mrs. Cross, will you hold Viola's arm for me?"

"Doctor," Erika said, "do you want the papoose?"

Maria Sanchez considered the device that would completely immobilize Viola's arms and legs. She looked into the girl's eyes and decided. "Viola, I think you can hold still for me, with Erika and your mom to help you. Do you think you can?"

"Yes. I can. I'm a big girl."

"I know you are. So let's try this way." With Mrs. Cross holding Viola's body and left arm and Erika holding her right arm firmly, Dr. Sanchez injected lidocaine in several spots around the girl's arm. Once the area was numb, she quickly placed eleven stitches in the girl's skin, then covered the area lightly with antibiotic cream and bandaged it to keep it clean. "How was that, Viola?"

"It wasn't too bad."

"Good." She reached into her pocket and pulled out a brightly colored piece of slick paper. "Do you like stickers?"

"Yes."

"Well, here's one for you." She handed the girl a two-inch round sticker and said, "This says 'Be Nice to Me, I Just Had Stitches.' "

"What do you say, Viola?" Mrs. Cross said.

"Thank you," Viola said, grinning.

"You're very welcome. Mrs. Cross, I'll give you the number for the health department so you can report this incident. Then they will contact us, and you'll come back tomorrow and four more times after that so Viola can get the medicine."

"Shots?" Viola said.

"Yes, but not bad ones. One tomorrow, then one three days after the first one, one a week after the first, one two weeks, and one four weeks later."

"I don't want all those shots."

"Viola," Dr. Sanchez said, "this is one place where you don't have a choice. This medicine will keep you from getting sick, and it's important that you have it."

Viola looked at her mother, who nodded. "Dr. Sanchez

is right, darling, but we'll make a nice day of it and maybe have lunch at Friendly's."

Not totally convinced but looking forward to hot dogs and a clown-face sundae, she nodded.

While Erika cleaned up the trash, Dr. Sanchez squeezed Viola's arm. "You were wonderful, Viola."

Suddenly Viola rolled onto her side and wrapped her small arm around the doctor's waist, squeezing gently. "Thank you, Doctor."

"Yes, thank you very much," Mrs. Cross said.

"You're very welcome. Just wait a few minutes and Erika will bring you the information from the health department, and we'll report it as well. Then I'll see you both tomorrow."

Dr. Sanchez opened the curtains and waved to Viola as she left the cubicle. Viola waved back, then blew a kiss at Dr. Sanchez's smiling face. "I love you," she whispered.

"Hugs, Viola," Dr. Sanchez said as she left to see her next patient.

Chapter 6

The roof of the market had been leaking for weeks, and Ramon Marquez, the store manager, had finally phoned his district manager to complain. "Just get three detailed proposals and quotes on the repairs and get back to me," the voice said, then hung up.

Ramon called several local roofing contractors and had one scheduled for that morning, one for the afternoon, and one for the following morning. He only hoped that the company's bureaucracy wouldn't hold things up long enough for the roof to collapse entirely. Shaking his head, he opened the market at 5:30 and surveyed the damage the previous night's rainstorm had done. "Not too bad," he said to Lois Carter, the first cashier to arrive. The wet spot in the ceiling over the cereal aisle had grown to about two feet in diameter, but the bucket Ramon had placed beneath it the previous evening was only half full. Since the dripping had stopped, Ramon dragged the bucket into the back of the store, emptied it, and stored it for the next rainstorm.

The market opened at 6:00 A.M. At about 8:10, several burly men invaded the supermarket. "We're from Apex Roofers," the largest of the men said.

Ramon looked from one to another. All the men were wearing stained and worn jeans and black T-shirts with APEX ROOFERS emblazoned on both the front and back. "Okay," he said. "What do you need from me?"

"Nothing. We've got everything we need in the truck. Just show us where the leaks are from the inside. We'll inspect the entire area then tell you what we find."

"Don't tell me. I need it all in writing. Just detail the problems, your proposed solutions, and give me a quote, all on paper. I wish I could make the decision but I can't. It has to go to the district."

"Okay," said the man who was obviously the leader. Ramon showed them the problem areas, then the three exited hastily leaving Ramon to calculate that, with all the company red tape, he probably wouldn't have his roof fixed for at least two months. Two months of buckets in the cereal aisle and God knows where else.

Outside, the three men unloaded their pickup truck and pulled the thirty-foot extension ladder off the side. They propped it against the south wall of the building and pulled the rope to raise the fly section. Old and frayed, the rope caught in a few places. "Damn," Tom Lakovitch said as he jiggled and pulled, catching his finger between two rungs as he extended the ladder. "Shit!" he said, shaking the pain from his finger, "I gotta replace this rope. Bob, remind me, will ya?"

"Sure," Tom's brother Bob said, pulling on his gloves. "But if you'd wear your gloves . . . "

"Get off my back," Tom said. "Just remind me about this rope."

"I reminded you last week and the week before."

"Just remind me tomorrow and shut up about it."

Les Gartner, a three-hundred-pound black man, was

used to the brothers' squabbles. "Let's just get this done," he said quietly. "We gotta get back to the Tomkins' house."

Still muttering, Tom and Bob finally got the ladder extended and the three men climbed onto the roof, three stories above the parking lot. For about thirty minutes they poked, prodded, lifted, and analyzed. "Not good," Tom muttered several times, shaking his head. "Not good at all."

"Gonna need a lot of work," Bob agreed. "Maybe the lower section is in better shape." He motioned to the rear of the building, which was only two stories tall.

"I doubt it," Tom said. "Looks like this is at least twenty-five years old." He pointed to a particular section. "Haven't done anything that way in years."

"Yeah," Bob said, nodding. "Let's go around back."

The three men climbed down the ladder. Remembering the trouble they had had extending it, Tom suggested, "Let's carry this bastard around back. I really don't want to lower the fly again." With Bob giving loud but useless directions, Tom and Les lifted the ladder, moved it away from the building, and started to lower it into a horizontal position for carrying. As the ladder came down, it touched the drop line that carried street current to the supermarket. Standing in a puddle left from the previous night's rain, all three men were electrocuted—rendered unconscious instantly.

David Boyd had stopped at the market's deli section on his way to work at the town highway department to grab a buttered roll for breakfast and a sandwich and a soda for lunch. As he left the market, he saw the three men collapse and heard the loud sparking from the place where the ladder touched the power lines. Without thinking, he ran over to help. As he stepped into the fringes of the puddle, he got a severe jolt of electricity and was thrown backward and knocked unconscious. Two other people followed him before the crowd realized that approaching the area was dangerous.

Inside the store, Ramon saw the lights flicker, then dim, and wondered what was wrong. He looked out the large glass front window and saw several people running toward the south side of the building. He dashed out the front door, saw the ladder still resting against the wires, and then spied the three unconscious roofers. "Stay back," he yelled. "That's a live wire. Everyone stay back."

"Get a stick," someone yelled, "and knock that ladder down."

"Use a rope," another cried.

"Do nothing!" Ramon yelled. "It's too dangerous. Just stay back." As he bolted back inside, he saw several men keeping the crowd about twenty feet from the puddle.

I was riding an early shift when the radio blared. "Fairfax Police to the ambulance. You're needed at the corner of Main and First, in the supermarket lot. We have a report of several people electrocuted."

"Make sure they called the power company," I said as Phil Ortiz, Steve Nesbitt, and I simultaneously jumped from the table.

Phil grabbed the mike. "Has the power company been notified?"

"Already done. They're on their way."

"10–4. We're en route with a four-minute ETA."

"10–4. Time is oh-nine-oh-five."

Steve had settled into the crew seat just inside the rear

section of the walk-through ambulance. I drove the rig out of the garage, then Phil closed the door and jumped into the shotgun seat. "Sounds awful, Joan. Should we get a second crew on standby?" he asked. Although he was nominally crew chief that morning, at that time he was a new EMT and still unsure of himself. Fortunately, he wasn't shy about asking for help.

We all knew that we could transport two or three non-critical victims but only one if the patient was critical. There's little enough room to work in the back of the rig. A second crew on standby in case they were needed sounded like good planning. "Might not be a bad idea," I said.

Phil grabbed the mike. Like all new riding members, he loved the feeling of talking on the radio. "45–01 to Fairfax Police."

"PD on. Go ahead, 45–01."

"Would you please page out for a standby crew and let us know how many injured we have as soon as you have an officer at the scene?"

"Sure will, –01. And I checked. The helicopter's not available." As we rolled toward the scene, we heard the pagers sound and the call go out. About a minute later, the dispatcher called us again. "FPD to unit responding to the supermarket."

"–01 on," Phil said.

"Officer at the scene requests that you expedite. Several victims. The power company just arrived and the power should be off by the time you arrive."

"10–4. Dispatch that second rig as soon as you have a crew and call for a Prescott rig as well since our third rig is down." Phil replaced the mike. "Joan," he said, "could you crew chief this one? I think I'll be in over my head."

"We can do it together. Just relax and remember your triage categories. Stable, unstable, critical, and black." Those in the black category were beyond any help. "We'll do what we can. That's all any of us can do. Yes?"

Phil nodded. "Yes."

We pulled into the parking lot and saw Officer Eileen Flynn waving us to one side. I parked and we got out as she ran up. "The power company will have the power off in about one minute. From what I can see, there are six people unconscious. All had contact with that puddle."

I quickly took in the ladder, the wires, and six unconscious people, all in or near the water. I looked at the crowd, now standing about fifty feet from the water.

"According to the store manager and several witnesses," Eileen said, "three of the injured were bystanders trying to help. The other three were contractors working on the roof."

Steve climbed out of the back of the rig with three crash bags, one for each of us.

"Hey, ambulance people," someone in the crowd shouted. "Aren't you going to help them?"

"Yeah," another voice yelled. "They're dying out there."

"We can't do anything until the power's shut off," Phil yelled. "We'll get to the victims as soon as we can."

"But they're dying."

"And these guys would be dying too," Eileen said in the direction of the crowd, "if they hadn't waited. Now keep your shirts on."

A hard-hatted power company employee ran up. "Power's off, guys. It's safe to go in now."

"Will you go first?" Steve said. "It's not that I don't trust you . . . "

"Sure," the power employee said, and walked in front of us to the first group of victims.

"Thanks," Steve said. "We'll take it from here."

"I'll take these three," I told Phil, indicating three men, still in the water, "while you check the two over there." I pointed and said, "Steve, see about that woman over there."

We separated. I approached the first man, a beefy middle-aged black man in jeans and a black T-shirt, crouched, and pressed my fingers against the man's neck just beside the Adam's apple. Nothing. I pressed against the other side and again found no pulse. Ordinarily I would have begun CPR, but with our limited manpower I needed to help those who had a chance. I moved to the second, then the third identically dressed man and got the same results.

I heaved a sigh, stood up, and moved to where Phil was assessing two more patients. "What have you got?" I asked, assuming scene control since this was an overwhelming situation even for an experienced EMT.

"That man's very scrambled, but I did a quick check and his vitals are stable and within normal range. This one's unconscious and his respirations are shallow and slow. Pulse is weak and thready. Yours?" I shook my head. "All *three*?" he asked. Again I shook my head.

"Eileen," I said, "get us the O_2 from your car and both of our oxygen duffels." Each duffel contained an oxygen cylinder and equipment to deliver it to our patients. Eileen, always helpful and very knowledgeable about EMS, nodded and headed toward the rig.

I moved to Steve's side. "How's your patient?"

"I need to bag her if we have the manpower. She's unconscious and her vitals are lousy."

Eileen had placed one oxygen duffel and a spare cylinder beside Phil and handed the other duffel to Steve. "We can manage if you're okay with Eileen to help you."

"Sure," Steve said, then, with Eileen's help, he began to care for the injured woman. As I returned to Phil a smartly dressed woman ran up to me. "I'm Dr. Julie Gilmore. I work at the ER in the trauma center."

"I thought you looked familiar," I said quickly. "Can you check those three over there? I couldn't find a pulse in any of them, but you can make it official." I couldn't pronounce so when the second crew arrived I would have to split my forces to work the codes unless a doctor decided they were beyond help.

"I'll check."

As she moved off to check the three contractors, I returned to Phil. "I would assume that these two were thrown when they contacted the puddle," I said. "See? The closest point they could have touched the live electricity is over there. In addition to the shock, we need to be careful about spinal injuries and broken bones." Since Phil was tending to his patient and the third victim was conscious, I could afford to take a moment and get organized. At this moment it was more important for me to have a clear overview of the situation than to treat.

I pointed to a crowd of people standing several yards away. "I need a few people who can help us. Any volunteers?" Several people walked toward me. "Great," I said. I pointed to a bearded man in his midforties. Since he was dressed in jeans, I hoped that he wouldn't mind getting them a bit dirty. "Can you kneel by this man's head and put your hands on either side? I'll show you how." He knelt down, put on the pair of latex gloves I handed him, and I showed him how to hold head stabilization on the groggy victim. "What's your name?"

"Mack."

"Okay, Mack. If you get too uncomfortable, let me know." I pointed to another man and asked, "Can you do the same thing for Phil's patient?"

"Sure. My name's Antonio." I handed him a pair of gloves and Antonio took head stabilization for Phil's patient, leaving Phil free to use the BVM to assist the patient's breathing. "As soon as you have some help," I said, hearing the siren from the approaching second ambulance, "do a better survey."

"Will do, Joan."

While I was talking, I attached a non-rebreather face mask to the third oxygen cylinder and placed the mask over my patient's face. I quickly ran my hands over the man's head and neck and, fortunately, found nothing but a slight bump at the back of his skull. As I checked his pulse with one hand, I pointed to a woman in the crowd who had said she would be able to help. "Go over there and see whether Steve and that officer need any help. Thanks." She walked off toward the group around the third patient.

I looked into the eyes of the still-groggy man and said, "Hi. My name's Joan. What's yours?" His pulse was strong and his breathing regular. While Mack continued to hold the man's head, I began to run my gloved hands slowly over my patient's chest, checking for broken ribs. Everything seemed to be intact.

After a long pause, the man said, "David. Boyd."

"Okay, David. Do you remember what happened?"

He pondered. "No. Not really," he said through the oxygen mask.

"Can you wiggle your fingers for me?" He did. "And your toes?" Those moved as well. I checked his pupils with my penlight and noted that they reacted appropriately.

"Well, it would seem that you got quite an electric shock." I pressed on his abdomen. "Does this hurt?"

"No. Not really."

I moved down to his legs. "Do you have any pain anywhere?"

"The back of my head." He paused. "My hands and feet are all tingly."

"I can imagine." I heard the second ambulance pull up and, in the distance, I heard the Prescott ambulance as well. Unfortunately, they wouldn't be bringing their paramedic since the call was out of their district.

Dr. Gilmore returned. "All three of them are beyond our help," she said softly. "I have a phone in my car so I'll make the notifications to the police and the county. Is there anything else I can do?"

"I think I'm okay. Would you check with Phil?" I nodded toward the still-green EMT.

"Sure." Dr. Gilmore crouched beside Phil and began to work with him checking out his patient. I returned to mine. I checked his hips and legs, then moved down to his feet.

"David," I said, "can you feel me touching your toes?" I squeezed the big toe on his right foot.

"Yes."

"Which one?"

"My right big toe. But it's still all tingly."

I squeezed his left foot. "And this?"

"My left baby toe."

"Good." I placed the palms of my hands against the soles of his feet and asked him to push down. The reactions were weak but even. I checked his hands, and when he squeezed my fingers his grip was steady. "Let me check your head again." I palpated the back of his skull and now found a larger lump. "Feels like you've got quite an egg on the back of your head. Any pain in your neck?"

"Not really. Just my head and that tingly feeling. I'm a bit fuzzed too."

"Just take it real easy for a few moments and we'll get you to the hospital." I stood up as Jack McCaffrey, who had arrived on the second rig, approached. "My guy can wait. Get Steve's patient and Phil's out of here first."

"Okay, Joan. We're loading Steve's into –01 and Phil's into –02. Can your guy come with either of them?"

"Since they're on their way anyway, I think I'd just as soon wait for Prescott." I could hear the siren in the distance, and it was getting closer. "They should be here in a moment and you'll need room to work. How are the others?"

"Both are still unconscious, but both seem to be breathing on their own. We're taking them to the trauma center."

"Good call. Since he seems not to be too badly off, I think mine can go to Fairfax General. That way we can keep the Prescott rig close to home."

"Okay." He pointed to the three men still in the puddle, now covered with blankets. "They're gone?"

"I'm afraid so," Dr. Gilmore pronounced. "What a lousy thing to happen. From what I understand, the ladder they were carrying must have touched the power lines. Unfortunately, it didn't fall when they did so current kept flowing. That's how the others got zapped, trying to help."

"Shit."

"Yeah."

We immobilized David to protect him from any additional damage and transported him to FGH. By the time we arrived, he was feeling much better. Fortunately for him, when he received the first shock he was close to the edge of the puddle and the jolt knocked him clear. He had a large lump on the back of his head but otherwise seemed none the worse for wear. He was seen in the ER and released a few hours later.

Phil, Steve, Jack, and I sat over coffee later at headquarters. "Both the woman and the man were admitted to the trauma center," Phil said, "but the doctors think they'll both be okay. She's got a broken leg and he might have a cervical fracture, but there's no neurological compromise. Glad we took spinal precautions. Thanks for the advice, Joan."

"We did good, guys," Steve said. "That was a tough situation, but it ran real well."

I took a deep breath and nodded. "It did go well. We did real good."

"I think this is the best sauce you've ever made," Hank Figueroa said to his wife, Eve. "Just fantastic."

Eve smiled. "Thanks," she said. "I read an article in a magazine about using alcohol in cooking so I used some red wine in this batch. I think it really added something."

Eve watched her husband twirl a gigantic forkful of spaghetti and stuff it into his mouth. "Great," he mumbled. "Fantastic." Hank, an electrician, was a large man who loved good food. Eve enjoyed taking the time to cook for him, despite her job as cashier at the local Home Depot and the fact that all their children were married and far away. She smiled as Hank smacked his lips. She loved it that he did as much as he could to encourage her to make some of her specialties, took seconds, and praised her constantly.

As Eve returned her attention to Tom Brokaw and the latest news from the Senate, Hank used his tablespoon to scoop up a large amount of meat and dump it on a slice of garlic bread. He took a large bite, chewed, and swallowed.

Most of the bite went down, but something stuck in his throat. He coughed but could not dislodge the object. "Something's stuck," he said, then coughed again.

"Are you choking?" Eve asked, not really concerned.

"I can breathe and all that," Hank said, clearing his throat, "but something's stuck. I can feel it." Eve got up, rounded the table, and pounded Hank on the back. "I don't think that's helping," Hank said, gagging and coughing. Eve then handed him his water glass and he took a swallow. That didn't help either.

"Let me call the doctor," Eve said.

"Not a chance," Hank said, heading for the bathroom, still trying to get the stuck object up.

In the bathroom he bent over the bowl, wondering whether he would vomit from his efforts to clear his throat. He remained in the bathroom for about five minutes, then returned to the dining room, still coughing.

"Dear," Eve said, "I think you need some help. I'm calling the doctor."

"It's 6:45. No one will be there anyway."

Eve reflexively glanced at her watch then looked back

at Hank. His face was red, his mouth open, his expression very distressed. "Then I'm calling the ambulance."

Although Hank wanted to protest again, he was beginning to wonder whether Eve wasn't right. Glad she was leaving him no choice, he sat, dropped his head between his knees, and continued to try to clear his airway.

I was in my kitchen with the microwave on but my ears perked up when the pagers sounded. Since I knew that the first rig was on another call, I pushed the STOP button so I could hear.

"Fairfax Police to all home units. An attendant is needed to meet the second ambulance for a person choking at unit 2A at Woodridge Condos. Any available unit please call in."

The Woodridge Condos were just down the road from my condos, so I pressed the speed dialer on my phone and told FVAC dispatcher Greg Horvath that I would respond to the scene. As I grabbed my purse and sprinted toward my car, I thought, It's going to be an RMA or a DOA. The person would either be better when I arrived and refuse medical attention, or he would be dead from lack of oxygen.

It took only thirty seconds for me to arrive at the scene. I grabbed my CPR mask from the glove compartment of my car and ran up the driveway. A middle-aged woman waited at the door. "He's in there," she said.

I found the man in the kitchen, sitting in a chair, his head between his knees. He was obviously breathing. "What's the problem?" I asked.

"I've got something in my throat," he said, coughing.

Relieved that I was not going to need to do CPR, I pushed the mask into my jacket pocket and keyed the mike on my FVAC portable. "45–24 to responding ambulance. Be advised that the patient is conscious and alert."

"10–4, Joan." I recognized Dave Hancock's voice.

Having told them that the situation wasn't critical, I returned my attention to my patient. "Can you talk to me without too much discomfort?" I asked.

"Yes," he said, his voice a bit hoarse.

"I'm Joan. And your name, sir?"

"Hank Figueroa."

"And I'm Eve. I'm his wife." She had been standing behind me watching. "He has something in his throat."

"Why do you think you have something in your throat? Can you feel it?"

Hank pointed just above his Adam's apple. "Right here."

"No trouble breathing?"

"None."

"Were you eating when this happened?"

"Yes. Spaghetti. What could get stuck from spaghetti?"

"I've got no clue." I heard the ambulance siren stop and soon Dave Hancock and Jill Tremonte arrived. We quickly took Hank's vital signs. "Your pulse and breathing are a bit fast," I told him, "probably from the excitement. Otherwise you're doing fine. Let's take you over to the hospital and let them check you out."

We drove, code 2, without any lights or siren, to FGH, where we left Hank and his wife to be examined by the staff.

A week later I saw the couple in the diner, having dinner. "Hi. Remember me? I was part of the ambulance crew that transported Hank last week."

"Sure. I remember," Eve said. "You're Joan."

"I guess everything turned out fine. What happened at the hospital?"

"Well," Hank said, putting his hamburger back onto his plate. "They stuck this thing down my throat and found the central rib of a bay leaf. Stuck. Wedged in my throat. They grabbed it out and presto, no more problem."

"A bay leaf?"

"Yup," Hank said. "From Evie's sauce."

"I think we'll eat out more now," Eve said. "The whole thing has got me spooked."

"It was a freak thing, Evie. You've got to keep cooking." He patted his large belly. "You've got to keep me healthy. This diner food's not nourishing." He took a big bite of his hamburger.

"Thanks so much for being there," Eve said. "You arrived so fast."

"You're welcome. That's what we're there for."

Hank swallowed a huge, partially chewed bite. "Yeah, thanks."

It was just a few minutes after 6:00 A.M. on Monday morning. "I got a roll of quarters. Can ya give me a ten for it?" The man speaking was a biker type, big, tattooed, bearded, and mean-looking. Behind him, the rest of the store was empty.

"Sure," Ben Knight said. Ben, just sixteen, worked the counter at Dunkin' Donuts before and after school. Mornings, the store usually got busy at around 6:30, when the commuters streamed in needing sustenance for their trip to the city. Ben had grown used to the mixed bag of doughnut eaters and coffee drinkers who wandered in and out. This guy, however, was stranger and meaner-looking than most. Ben glanced out of the large front window into the early-morning darkness and saw the man's large purple Honda motorcycle parked in the handicapped space adjacent to the store. "Nice bike," he said.

"Yeah," the big man replied.

Ben knew it was company policy not to make change, but he wasn't about to argue. He punched the keys to open the register and pulled out a ten-dollar bill. As he closed the register, he felt a sudden pain in the side of his face under his ear and down his neck and he fell backward. The last thing he saw was the big guy opening the register and scooping out the bills.

By the time Jeff Sunderberg, morning manager, walked out of the back of the doughnut shop, the robber had already gone. Unaware of what had happened, Jeff walked past the display of dozens of kinds of freshly baked doughnuts, wondering where Ben had gotten to. "Hey, Ben. We need another pot of coffee." Just then Jeff found the young man at the far end of the counter, lying in a pool of blood. With shaking hands he dialed 911.

Ed and I were just getting dressed when the pagers sounded. For some reason, FVAC had been having difficulty covering early-morning calls, particularly on Mondays. "I can't go," Ed said. "I've got that dentist appointment at 7:30." Ed had been suffering with a broken tooth since the previous Saturday evening.

"I've got a manuscript deadline at the end of this week," I said. "Let's see what they need and who's around."

"FPD to all home units. The ambulance is needed at Dunkin' Donuts for the victim of an assault. The officer at the scene says the scene is safe and asks that you expedite."

Ed and I exchanged looks. "Let's take two cars," Ed said. "I can't go to the hospital with you but I can help you at the scene."

I pressed the speed-dial button on my phone and notified the police that I was responding. I didn't mention Ed since he wouldn't be part of the crew.

"Thanks, Joan," Mark Thomas said. "Seems the kid working there was slashed real bad."

I hung up and filled Ed in as we ran toward our cars.

When we arrived, the Dunkin' Donuts' parking lot was filled with police cars. Since it was only a few blocks from my condo, Ed and I were the first EMS units to arrive.

Will McAndrews ran up. "Kid's bleeding bad," he said as I pulled on gloves and got my crash kit from my trunk. "The perp's long gone. If you can, get any information from the kid that might help us."

"Will do," I said.

Together Ed and I entered the chaotic scene and were quickly waved behind the counter. I had never seen so much blood. As I knelt beside the young man, the source of the bleeding became obvious. He had a gaping slash wound that began under his left ear and ran down the side of his neck, then angled toward his Adam's apple. I placed my gloved hand over the wound, applying just a bit of pressure to slow the bleeding. I opened my crash kit, grabbed at a handful of 4 × 4s, and tore them open. I quickly realized, however, that they wouldn't be suffi- cient to cover the wound. "Ed," I said, "this gauze isn't going to be enough. Get me something bigger. And I'll need an occlusive dressing."

As I bent over the victim, Ed unwrapped a large trauma dressing, then carefully folded the heavyweight plastic packaging, inside out, into a flat pad. This airtight, occlusive dressing would keep air from entering the cut jugular vein. Without it a bubble of air could be sucked into that large vein. The resulting air bubble would go straight to the heart and act like a blood clot, stopping the heart and killing the patient.

The boy was covered with blood from the chest up, and I had no idea how I was going to hold the dressing in place. Tape would never stick and I couldn't wrap anything totally around the boy's neck. As Ed prepared the dressing, I bent over. "Can you hear me?"

The boy moaned.

"What's his name?" I asked, looking up.

"Ben," someone said. "His name's Ben."

"Ben. I'm Joan and we're taking care of you." The boy moaned again.

"Do you remember getting cut?" Another moan.

"Can you tell me anything about the person who did this?" Ed handed me the plastic pad and I lifted my hand and pressed it against the wound. I took note of the fact that the blood was darker colored and flowing, not spurting. The boy's carotid artery was probably all right, but he was losing a great deal of blood from a partially cut or severed jugular vein.

"Biker," the boy whispered.

"Ed, I need another dressing and a roll of gauze." I tried to recall the picture in the textbook of the figure-eight bandage that might hold enough pressure on the wound to slow the bleeding. "Will," I said to the officer who stood behind me, "the boy said 'biker.' "

"Great. See whether you can get a description," he said.

"Ben," I said, adding another layer of thick gauze over the soaked one already in place, "can you tell us anything that might help the cops get the guy who did this?" As I continued to hold the dressing against the wound, I heard the siren of the approaching ambulance.

His eyes remained closed, his voice soft. But with my face near his mouth I could hear the word "dagger."

"Dagger?" I asked.

"Arm."

"A tattoo? Just make one sound if that's right."

Ben moaned once.

"Will," I said, "Ben says the guy had a tattoo of a dagger on his arm."

"He said the guy was a biker," Will said. "Did he have a motorcycle? Did the kid see it?"

"Honda," the boy whispered. With a small smile he added, "Purple."

"He says the guy had a purple Honda."

"Great job, kid," Will said. "We'll catch him for you."

Ben sighed, then was silent. As the ambulance and crew arrived, Ed handed me a roll of wide gauze. "Backboard and stretcher," Ed said to Linda Potemski and Nick Abrams. Linda handed Ed the crash kit and oxygen, then she and Nick returned to the rig for the equipment. "And a blanket," I called.

I took the roll of gauze and, starting at the bandage on Ben's neck, wrapped a layer around the neck then across the opposite shoulder and under that arm, back up, again across the shoulder, and around the injured side of his neck, forming a figure eight. That put some pressure on the injury but did not surround the boy's throat. As I wound several more circuits, Ed set up the oxygen and quickly put the non-rebreather mask to Ben's face. Now the boy would be breathing 100 percent oxygen. He was beginning to shiver and he was sweating profusely.

"Ed, check his radial pulse. He's diaphoretic and cold."

I watched Ed try to find a pulse. He shook his head. "BP must be too low for that. Do you want to MAST?"

The inflatable military antishock trousers would put pressure on Ben's lower body, increasing the circulation to vital organs. Although there was controversy over their use, MAST was state protocol and it might help. "Yes," I said, "but let's do it in the rig." I found the carotid pulse on the uninjured side of Ben's neck and noted that the beating was very rapid.

The four of us half rolled, half lifted Ben onto the backboard and placed him on his uninjured side and strapped him down. Then we lifted him onto the stretcher and arranged the mechanism to raise the boy's feet and increase his upper-body circulation. "Have you got enough help? I'll stay if you need me," Ed said.

"Go, Ed. We're fine."

With the help of several others, we lifted the stretcher into the rig and sped off, lights and siren toward the trauma center. In the ambulance, Linda and I struggled to get the MAST onto the boy's lower body. "Nick," I yelled through the window to the cab, "call this in. We're a bit busy back here."

I heard Nick stop the siren and tone the code for the trauma center. While waiting for the hospital to answer, Linda and I succeeded in getting the MAST onto Ben's legs and lower abdomen. Linda attached the air hoses and rhythmically pressed the foot pump. I returned to Ben's head and put a bit more pressure on the dressings over his wound.

I listened to Nick's report. "We are en route with a teenage boy, a victim of a slashing. The injury is to his neck. We have an occlusive dressing in place and . . . "

I yelled at him, "MAST applied. Being inflated now."

" . . . MAST being inflated now. Our ETA is about five minutes."

"Do you have the patient's vitals?"

"Vitals?" Nick yelled.

"No got," I yelled back.

"Vitals are not available at this time," Nick said into the mike.

There was a moment of silence, then the voice from the trauma center said, "The doctor needs vitals."

I heard and yelled to Nick, "Tell him pulse rapid, breathing fast and shallow. BP below eighty." I could estimate his blood pressure from the lack of a radial pulse. I heard Nick relay the information to the trauma center.

"The doctor says he needs accurate vitals."

I looked at Linda. "It's not as if they'll change the first thirty seconds of treatment depending on what his vitals are," I said. "Then they'll take their own set. We're a bit busy here." I kept moderate pressure on Ben's neck wound while Linda continued to inflate the MAST.

"They must have a new doctor who wants all the i's dotted and the t's crossed," Linda said. "The first week is the worst."

"Yeah. He wants vitals and the people in hell want ice water," Nick muttered, clearly furious. He keyed the mike. "Look, Doctor. We'll give you what we've got when we get it." He released the key.

"Thank you, 45–01. We'll be expecting you. St. Luke's clear."

"Phew," I said to Linda, raising an eyebrow. "I guess that said it."

When we arrived at the trauma center, I was glad to see that Ben's condition appeared to be improving. His breathing was easing and the new dressing I had added to the ones on his injury hadn't yet soaked through. We wheeled the stretcher through the ER doors and were directed to trauma 2. "I wonder what's in trauma 1," I muttered.

"Bad car wreck," Erika Morely said. "Dr. Gilmore's been in there for half an hour."

As we transferred the patient to the trauma stretcher, a young doctor bustled into the room. "Is this the neck injury?"

"This is Ben," I answered, a large chip on my shoulder. It always annoys me when a person is treated as "an injury." "He has a slash wound that begins just below the ear and continues to just beside the Adam's apple. I'd estimate about four inches long, superficial for about half of that, deeper over the jugular vein area."

"That was a poor report we got over the radio," the doctor said.

Nick took a breath and gritted his teeth. "I was polite," he hissed.

As I started to say something, Dr. Gilmore arrived. "Not in front of the patient," she snapped.

She was right, and I swallowed my retort.

We left the room, made up the stretcher, and waited for a few minutes to speak to both doctors. As Ben, with three IV lines refilling his fluids and blood en route from the blood bank, was wheeled toward CT scan, Dr. Gilmore, followed by the doctor who had been involved in the radio transmissions, approached us.

"Nice job, guys," Dr. Gilmore said. "That occlusive dressing may have saved his life. And great bandaging job."

"Thanks," I said.

"I'm Dr. Warren," the other doctor said, "and I'm sorry about that radio business. I guess you were a bit busy out there."

"Yeah," Nick said, "we were."

"I got a bit carried away," Dr. Warren continued. "Erika said to just skip it. I guess she was right."

"We all just want what's best for our patients," Dr. Gilmore said, smiling warmly at the three of us. "Dr. Warren's a second-year resident and it's his first week here. No one else was available." She turned to the new resident. "And listen to your nurses. It's a good lesson. They usually know what's needed." She grinned. "You'll learn quickly enough, and it was a small thing." Dismissed, Dr. Warren hurried away.

"He's a bit green and wet behind the ears, but he's actually a really good doctor. He just needs field experience." She cocked her head to one side. "I may ask him to ride with you guys for a few shifts. It would do him lots of good to see how it is 'out there.' "

"Sure, Doc," Nick said.

"By the way," Dr. Gilmore said, "what was it you said there at the end?"

"It's the punch line of an old joke. A six-year-old girl and a six-year-old boy are standing together on the playground. The previous evening, the little boy had seen an old George Raft movie and now the boy is flipping a quarter saying, over and over, 'I *want* what I *want* when I *want* it.'

"Finally sick of it, the little girl says, 'I'll *give* you what I've *got* when I *get* it.' "

We all laughed and we left the trauma center. Two days later I read the article in the local paper.

Man Accused of Slashing

A man identified as Peter Franklin, of northern California, was arrested yesterday and accused of the slashing of a Dunkin' Donuts employee. Ben Knight, 16, of Poplar Street, Fairfax, was cut from his left ear to the center of his neck, a wound requiring more than 100 stitches. Despite his serious injury, Mr. Knight was able to give enough information to the police to allow them to capture the alleged slasher only a few hours later.

Mr. Knight, interviewed at his home the day after the incident, stated that the man first asked for change, slashed him with what he assumes was a box cutter, then emptied the cash register. He thanked the ambulance crew and the hospital staff for their quick action in saving his life.

Franklin is being held without bail in the county jail pending arraignment.

Chapter 7

Dan Jamison was lying on a ten-foot-square raft in the middle of Wanacosa Lake, enjoying the warmth of the early-morning sun. He could hear the echoing *pweet-pweet-pweet* call of a cardinal and the *peter-peter-peter* of a tufted titmouse from the fifty-year-old trees that ringed the lake. Although it meant getting up an hour earlier than he had to, Dan often walked over to the Wanacosa Lake beach early in the morning during the warm weather and swam out to the raft. He would relax in the sun for ten or fifteen minutes before swimming back to the beach. Then he would take a quick shower and begin his thirty-minute commute to work. It was so peaceful on the lake on this unusually warm, late-spring morning that he wished that he could stay longer.

Glancing toward the beach, he saw another early-morning swimmer enter the water and begin to paddle toward the raft. He was disappointed. Dan didn't really feel like socializing, and he resented having his morning solitude interrupted. Oh, well, he thought, it's a public beach. He idly watched the swimmer, a middle-aged woman, approach the raft. The woman was attractive, with dark gray-streaked hair, but her face appeared to be drawn. She seemed to be having some difficulty swimming. The woman reached the raft, climbed the ladder, and sat down heavily. Her face was pale and her breathing rapid as she clutched her left shoulder. "Are you all right?" Dan asked.

"I guess so," she replied uncertainly. "I'm just out of breath."

"Did you hurt your shoulder?"

"No. I don't think so," she answered. "But it hurts." Suddenly the woman's eyes widened. "I can't breathe." She gasped, then fell face forward onto the raft. Her body convulsed for a few seconds, then she was still.

Dan scrambled over to the woman and turned her onto her back. Her eyes were wide open, but they were staring sightlessly at the sky. Dan was panic-stricken, feeling helpless and alone. He searched the empty beach wildly and began shouting for help. He looked down at the woman, who was absolutely still and did not appear to be breathing. Dan thought of the CPR training that he had had a few months earlier and tried to remember what to do. He had had to take the class to coach his son's Little League team, but he'd paid only minimal attention. He never thought that he would actually have to do compressions or ventilations. Dan remembered his CPR instructor's advice: If you feel panicky, stop everything you're doing and take a deep breath.

Dan closed his eyes, took a deep breath, and thought of the CPR procedures. Open the airway and look, listen, and feel, he remembered. He tipped the woman's head back, put his ear next to her mouth, and looked at her chest. There was no sound, he could feel no breath against his cheek, and her chest was not moving.

Give two breaths. He recalled that he should use a pocket mask or mouth shield when giving breaths for artificial ventilation, but here on the raft that was not an option. Dan pinched the woman's nose closed with his left hand and blew into her mouth. He repeated the procedure again, then slid the middle finger of his right hand to the side of her neck. Dan could not find a pulse. The woman was in cardiac arrest. Dan knew that unless he began CPR, the woman would be beyond any help within a few minutes.

Dan looked toward the shore and saw a man watching him from a window of a house next to the beach. "Call an ambulance," Dan shouted, waving his arms. The man didn't seem to understand. "Call the police," Dan tried again, shouting as loud as he could. The man disappeared from the window. Dan didn't know whether he had understood him or not, but there was no one else around. He knew what he had to do now. He positioned himself over the woman's chest, felt for the notch at the bottom of her breastbone with his right hand, positioned his left hand over her chest, covered it with his right, and began compressing her chest. One-and-two-and-three . . . he counted, praying that someone had been alerted to what was happening.

Prescott Police Officer Roy Zimmerman had just begun his duty tour and was patrolling one of Prescott's scenic but curvy back roads. On a pretty, warm late-spring morning like this, what could go wrong? he thought.

Prescott had once been a summer vacation area. Fifty years earlier, the houses around Wanacosa Lake had been unheated summer cottages. Vacationers from the city had referred to the area as the country. Now, although still quite rural, Prescott was a suburb of the city and people preferred to travel farther away for their vacations. So most of the summer cabins had been enlarged, heated, and converted to year-round homes. Still, between the Fourth of July and Labor Day, lots of people, including day visitors from the city came to "the country" to have fun and get into trouble. Well, we should have a few more weeks of peace, Roy thought as he crested the hill overlooking Wanacosa Lake.

"GRQ-325 to 703," Roy's radio blared.

Roy unclipped the mike from its holder and pressed the key. "703," he said.

"Check Wanacosa Lake beach. We have a report of someone having some sort of a problem out on the raft."

"10–4. What's my priority?"

"Better make it priority 3." Since the dispatcher didn't know what the problem was, he was taking no chances. Rather than obeying the traffic rules as code 2 driving would indicate, Roy would use his police car's emergency lights and siren to rush to the beach area.

Roy replaced the mike, flipped several of the switches on his dash, and, lights flashing and siren wailing, headed toward the beach.

As the police car pulled up to the fence, Roy looked out toward the raft. He could see a man kneeling over a body. The man's arms were extended and his shoulders were rhythmically moving up and down. One glance was enough to tell Roy exactly what was going on. Shit, he thought, what a place to have to do CPR. He grabbed his mike. "703 to 325," he barked.

"325 is on."

"It looks like someone's doing CPR out on the raft. Get me a 10–12 and dispatch Prescott Fire and the Rescue Squad. And tell them we'll need a boat." The request for a 10–12 would bring backup units to the scene.

"10–4, 703."

Roy switched his mike to the PA setting. "Hang on out there," his amplified voice boomed. "Help is on the way." The man on the raft paused in his compressions just long enough to wave an acknowledgment.

Roy ran to the back of his cruiser, grabbed his portable oxygen tank from the trunk, and ran to the lifeguard's boat on the beach. "Damn," he said, looking down into the small craft. There were no oars. Roy threw the oxygen tank into the boat, dragged the boat into the water, then pushed it in the direction of the raft as hard as he could and jumped in. Moving from one side to the other, he paddled with his hands, until, after what seemed like hours, he reached the floating platform. Not taking time to secure the boat, which would be useless for transporting the patient, Roy threw the oxygen tank onto the raft and climbed on.

Dan, who looked nearly exhausted, was no longer doing chest compressions but was still doing artificial ventilations—blowing into the woman's mouth. "She had no pulse after she collapsed," he reported between breaths, "but she has a faint one now."

"Good work, guy," Roy said. "Give me a few seconds to set up the oxygen and I'll relieve you." Roy opened the oxygen tank carrying case, pulled out the tank, opened the main valve, and adjusted the oxygen flow to fifteen liters per second. He then unwrapped a BVM, hooked it up to the oxygen, and moved to the woman's head. "Why don't you take a break," he said to Dan as he got ready to force high-flow oxygen into the woman's lungs.

With great relief, Dan moved to the side. Like all Prescott Police officers, Roy was well trained in CPR. He felt for a carotid pulse and placed his cheek next to the woman's mouth to check for breathing. "You're right," he said to Dan. "She does have a pulse. She's lucky you were here to start CPR."

Suddenly the woman's chest expanded as she took a deep breath. "She's breathing," Dan yelled.

"Hold on," Roy said as both men watched. The breath was not followed by another. "It's what's called agonal breathing," Roy said. "It's not enough to keep her alive." He fitted the BVM mask over the woman's face and began to squeeze the bag.

By now the air was alive with the wails of approaching police and rescue vehicles. Within ten minutes the Prescott Fire Department had its rescue boat in the water with two EMTs aboard. Less than ten minutes later, the woman was in the ambulance en route to Fairfax General Hospital under the care of paramedic Hugh Washington and Prescott EMTs Brenda Frost and Sally Walsh. By the time they arrived at the ER, while Sally and Brenda ventilated, Hugh had drawn several vials of blood for the hospital to test and established an IV line in the woman's arm. As they pulled into the bay, the woman began to breathe on her own.

My Prescott crew and I had delivered a delightful woman who had been complaining of flulike symptoms to the emergency room at FGH, and I was standing outside in the warm spring air as the second Prescott ambulance pulled into the bay. The back doors opened and I helped the crew pull out the stretcher and lower it to the ground. As we wheeled the woman into the emergency room, Brenda told me what had happened. "I'd never have believed that anyone had a chance under those circumstances, Ed. On a raft."

"Me either," I said. "You mean some guy did CPR on that raft in the middle of Wanacosa Lake?"

"And saved her life too."

The woman moaned and opened her eyes. "What happened?" she asked.

"We'll let the doctors figure that out," Hugh said, "but I would say that an angel just landed on your shoulder and saved your life."

The doctors would, of course, have to discover the cause of her heart problem and take appropriate steps to prevent a recurrence of her sudden death, but, in all probability, she would live to swim again, thanks to Dan Jamison and the CPR course he had to take.

Young people sometimes think of the elderly as frail, gentle grandparent types. It isn't always so.

The call had come in that an elderly woman who fell was having difficulty breathing. We could hear her screams and moans as soon as we opened the door of the Rutlandt Nursing Home. As crew chief, I was leading, carrying a trauma kit and oxygen. Steve Nesbitt and Tim Babbett followed, pulling the stretcher on which we had placed a long backboard, collars, and straps.

We walked down the long corridor, sidestepping and twisting to avoid colliding with the wheelchair- and walker-bound residents who filled the corridor. At the end of the hallway, a group of nursing home staff members and residents were gathered around someone lying on the floor next to the corridor wall. The group parted as we approached and I could see a very large woman who lay on her back, screaming "Oh! The pain. I can't stand the pain!"

I turned to Syl Farmington, one of Rutlandt's nurses. "What happened?" I asked.

"Hi, Ed. She took a fall, but I haven't been able to find out where she's hurt. She's been yelling like this since she fell."

"What the hell are you all standing around for?" the woman screamed. "I'm dying. Why the hell don't you do something for me? Give me oxygen. I need oxygen."

"Did anyone see her fall?" I asked.

"Oh, God, the pain," the woman screamed.

"Yeah, I saw her go down," Syl replied. "She kind of slid down against the wall. She didn't seem to fall very hard and I really didn't think that she was hurt."

"You're an idiot," the woman screamed. "Can't you see that I'm hurt?"

"Do you know what made her fall?" I asked.

Syl looked at another of the Rutlandt nurses, then turned back to me. "Well"—Syl hesitated—"she sort of tried to push another woman out of her way, but she lost her balance and fell down."

"That bitch was walking slowly just to spite me," the woman shrieked. "Now look what she did to me. She ought to be in jail."

I suddenly remembered an ambulance call I had responded to a few weeks earlier. A frail ninety-two-year-old had been pushed by another woman and had broken her arm. I had learned since that the woman, Mary Louise Grant, had been responsible for a number of injuries at Rutlandt over the past few years. It seemed that she liked to barrel down the corridors with her walker, pushing people out of her way.

"Is this Mary Louise Grant?" I asked.

"The one and only," Syl replied. "We all call her Mary."

"Glad you're in charge of this one," Steve muttered under his breath, his words inaudible to anyone but me. "I think I'd kill her."

"Yeah, right," I murmured back.

"It hurts so bad," Mary screamed. "Why did this have to happen to me?"

I knelt next to her. "Where are you hurt?" I asked.

"All over. I hurt all over. Oh, God, do something you idiot."

I examined Mary thoroughly while she continued to scream, curse, and bemoan her fate. She shrieked and complained of tenderness wherever I touched her, but I could find no evidence of injury. Aside from what appeared to be point tenderness over every inch of her body, there was no swelling, deformation, or discoloration anywhere. Her vital signs were within normal limits, and she had good movement, sensation, and pulses in her hands and feet.

"I can't find anything wrong with you, Mary," I said, "but we'll take you over to the hospital and get you checked out. Okay?"

"What do you mean, you can't find anything wrong with me? What the fuck good are you? Where the hell did you go to medical school?" she yelled. "Oh, God. Why me? Why me? I need oxygen."

"I'm not a doctor, Mary," I replied. "I'm an emergency medical technician and it is not my job to diagnose what's wrong with you. All I can do is take you to the hospital and tell them what I've found. And I'm not going to give you oxygen. With all your screaming, you're hyperventilating. You're getting too much oxygen. I need you to calm down and slow your breathing down."

"You're not a doctor?" She glared at me. "Then get the fuck out of here. I want a goddamn doctor, not an emergency mechanic."

It was becoming obvious to Syl that my patience was beginning to wear thin. She stepped in. "Mary," she said, "these people are trying to help you. Let them take you to the hospital so you can be examined by a doctor."

"I don't want their goddamn help and I'm not going to no hospital. Oh, God, why did this happen to me?"

I decided to try the tough approach. "Look, Mary," I said in an angry tone that I did not have to fake. "You are keeping an emergency ambulance out of service that might be needed by someone else with a medical emergency. I am recommending that you go to the hospital and I'm advising you that refusing to go may cause serious harm to you. Since you claim that your neck and back hurt, we will have to immobilize you completely on a board in order to transport you to the hospital. Of course, we cannot force you to go with us, but if you refuse to go, we will ask you to sign a release stating that you are refusing to be transported to the hospital. Then we will leave. Do you understand what I have told you?"

"I'm not gonna lay on a goddamn board and I'm not gonna sign nothing."

"Okay," I said, turning over my PCR and handing it to Syl. "Syl, if you and the other nurse would please sign as witnesses that Mary is refusing transport, we'll get our ambulance back into service. There doesn't seem to be any way to convince her to go."

"All right, all right," Mary suddenly said. "I'll go

in your goddamn ambulance. But no fucking board under me."

"Sorry, Mary," I replied, "you have no choice in the matter. If you want to be transported by us, you will have to let us do our job the way you are best protected from further injury." It wasn't that I wanted to torture the woman, although the thought was tempting. Her belligerence might just lead her to sue us if anything went wrong so I was going to play this one strictly by the book.

With much wailing and swearing, but no further resistance, Mary allowed Tim, Steve, and me to apply a cervical collar to her neck, fully immobilize her on a longboard, and transport her to Fairfax General. The last thing we heard as we wheeled the empty stretcher out of the hospital was Mary screaming at the emergency room physician. "You call yourself a fucking doctor? Where the hell did you get your goddamn medical degree? I need some goddamn oxygen."

It was Memorial Day weekend. For the past fifteen years, Harvey Rosen's Memorial Day barbecue had been a Floral Court development tradition. All the neighbors were invited and everyone always had a great time. In the past, the weather had always cooperated.

This year, however, rain was forecast for the entire three-day weekend, and it looked like the barbeque would be a washout. Sunday evening, however, on the eleven o'clock news, Rick Steele predicted that the rain would stop early Monday morning and that the holiday would be sunny and unusually hot. "Yes!" Harvey shouted, raising his fist in the air and bringing it down sharply. Harvey turned off the TV, snuggled up to his wife, June, who was already asleep, and drifted off, thankful that he had opened the pool and not canceled the barbecue.

By 11:00 A.M. the sun was shining and steam was rising from the wet grass of Harvey's backyard. The yard had grown progressively smaller in the years since the kids left home, as the adjoining forest crept toward his house. After all, what did he and June need with a big backyard? But it was still big enough to accommodate the neighbors at his Memorial Day better-this-year-than-ever-before barbecue. Harvey called a few of his neighborhood buddies that morning to assure them that the barbecue was a "go."

"Great news, Harve," Bruce Wilcox, his next-door neighbor said. "I'm really looking forward to it. I'll be over early to help out."

Harvey now grinned in anticipation. The coolers were filled with beer and soft drinks. Although most of his friends liked good ordinary beer like Bud, he had picked up some of the new microbrewery beers that were getting so popular. Some of the darker beers were not bad, he thought, but how could anyone drink something like that German apfel-honig weissbier? Oh well, Harvey thought, there's no accounting for foreign tastes. He didn't realize that the sweetened fermented wheat beer had been produced in a Brooklyn microbrewery.

The refrigerator was filled with marinating chicken, hamburger patties, and franks just waiting for the fire to get hot. Harvey dumped some charcoal into the bottom of the grill, sprinkled starter fluid onto it, and tossed in a lighted match to ignite the fluid. He watched the starting fluid flare up, then turned and went into the kitchen to help June prepare dips for the chips and veggies. Having barbecued so often, Harvey knew exactly how much fluid to use to start the charcoal.

Fifteen minutes later, Harvey came out and looked at the charcoal, expecting to see white edges as the briquettes began to burn. But there was nothing. The grill was cold. Shit, Harvey thought, the bag of charcoal had been outside during all that rain. Although it had been sheltered from the worst of the downpour, it must have absorbed a lot of moisture. Harvey opened the can of starter fluid again, poured a large amount of fluid on the charcoal, tossed in a lighted match, and watched everything ignite with a *whoosh*. He watched as the flame died down, then he stirred the briquettes, encouraging them to burn. Some of the edges began to catch, but then they went out without spreading to the centers of the briquettes. Damn, Harvey thought, people will be coming soon and they'll be hungry. This charcoal is just too wet. For the third time, he opened the can of starter fluid and started to pour it onto the charcoal, just as Bruce came around the corner of the house.

"Hey, Harve," Bruce called, "how's it going? What can I do to help?"

Harvey turned to greet his neighbor just as a tiny charcoal ember ignited the stream of starter fluid that he was pouring. During the second that Harvey turned toward Bruce, the flame flashed up the stream and the can became a ball of fire in his hands. Harvey was still looking at Bruce when the shock of pain caused him to release the can, which bounced on the ground, spraying his legs and shoes with burning fluid. He looked down and saw that his legs were burning and he was standing in a pool of fire. He started to run, screaming with pain and terror. Suddenly he felt himself fall to the ground and roll over and over. Bruce had knocked him down, grabbed a large towel from a nearby lawn chair, and rolled him in it. Then Bruce rolled Harvey's blanket-wrapped body over and over in the grass.

Twenty-year-old Jill Tremonte and I were lounging in front of headquarters watching the steam rise from the wet pavement. The humidity and heat were reminiscent of August rather than the end of May. It was early in Jill's career at Fairfax and, although she had done well in her EMT class and had earned a grade of 92 percent on her state EMT exam, she had not yet been crew chief— the EMT in charge—of a serious call.

Different emergency response organizations have different systems for determining who is in charge of a call. Some, like Fairfax, maintain duty rosters that specify the crew chief. In others, like Prescott where no daytime crews are on duty, the first EMT at the scene or the first to call in when the pagers sound automatically becomes the crew chief and is expected to accompany the patient to the hospital. This assures continuity of care.

Despite the fact that she had done well in her EMT training, Jill was still reluctant to be crew chief. "I don't know whether I'm ready for that kind of responsibility," she told me as we sat on the redwood picnic table. "Like yesterday." She had told me about the call she had responded to the previous day.

On the Sunday of the holiday weekend, there had been few people available and the dispatcher had paged out three times for an EMT to cover a personal injury automobile accident. Receiving no response, he announced that he was about to call the neighboring Prescott Rescue

Squad for mutual aid. Jill decided to take the risk and called in as EMT and crew chief.

The accident had been a relatively minor one, and there had been only one patient who had been complaining of neck and back pain. Jill had completed her examination of the patient and had asked her crew to bring over spinal immobilization equipment when a car with green light flashing pulled up. Fred Stevens, a long-time Fairfax member, jumped out of the car and ran over. When Jill hesitated, Fred took over command of the scene. Jill, thoroughly intimidated, stood off to the side while Fred directed the immobilization and extrication of the patient. Then he did the paperwork, totally ignoring Jill, who was nominally crew chief for the call.

Now, standing in front of the firehouse, Jill finished telling me the story and was angrily complaining about Fred's behavior. "He all but pushed me out of the way," she said. "He had no right to take over that call. I knew what I was doing."

"Well," I replied, "if you want to remain in control of an emergency situation, you're going to have to be more assertive. Fred is a good EMT but he's very aggressive. He's also been around a long time and, by habit, he just takes over. Don't get me wrong. He's great to have with you on a bad call, and he'll back off if you let him know that you're crew chief. You don't learn it in your EMT class, but it's important to remain in charge of your patient. The crew chief has to make the ultimate decisions about what treatment will be given."

I've taught dozens of EMT classes and this was a lesson Jill needed to learn. "Sometimes cops, nurses, or even ordinary bystanders will try to second-guess you and tell you what to do. But your name is what goes on the bottom of the prehospital care report. That means that if someone decides to file a lawsuit, you're the one who will be sued. So you'd better be sure that you're the one who makes the decisions about your patient or that you agree with any suggestions that someone else at the scene makes. Listen to suggestions, but treat your patient in whatever way you, and only you, think is best."

"I understand what you're saying, but I'm not like that. It feels pushy."

"Maybe it is a bit pushy, but that's how things get done." I patted her knee, noting that she was about the age of my oldest daughter. Since our insurance company had laid down the law and told us that no one under twenty-one was allowed to drive, she was crew chief today. "I remember one call a long time ago. It was a motorcycle accident and I was crew chief. When we got to the scene, a guy with a stethoscope draped over his neck was kneeling over the patient. He was very authoritative and barked orders to me and my crew. I thought he was a doctor and he certainly seemed to know what he was doing, so I did what he told me to do. Fortunately, he really did know what he was doing and the motorcyclist, who had a broken leg, was well treated. But I later found out that the man who had taken charge of the scene so authoritatively was a veterinarian."

"You're right," Jill said with a sigh. "But I'm not a very aggressive person, and—"

Jill and I were startled by the sound of the klaxon, which signaled an emergency call. "Fairfax PD to the ambulance."

We walked into the building and Jill picked up the mike. "Ambulance on."

"The rig is needed at 471 Oak Hill," the police

dispatcher said. "That's in the Floral Court development. It's a fifty-four-year-old male with severe burns."

I turned to Jill. "You can't drive so I will and you can be the EMT. That way we can respond immediately and have an attendant meet us at the scene. Okay?"

Jill got that deer-in-the-headlights look. "This sounds like a bad one," she said. "I'm not sure I can handle it."

"I'll be with you at the scene," I reassured her. "I'll back you up if you need help and I'll make suggestions, but I won't take over. You're well trained and you'll do fine."

"Okay." She keyed the mike. "45–01 is responding to 471 Oak Hill in Floral Court for a man with severe burns. Please page out for an attendant to meet us at the scene."

"Will do. Your time is eleven fifty-seven."

"And put the helicopter on standby."

"10–4," the police dispatcher said.

"Good thinking," I told Jill as we went toward the ambulance. Because of the location of Floral Court, the regional burn center at St. Luke's was about twenty-five minutes away by ground ambulance. A serious burn patient should be transported by helicopter if at all possible.

As I nosed the ambulance out of the building, I could hear the pager tones on the radio. "Fairfax Police to all home units. An attendant is needed to meet 45–01 at 471 Oak Hill for a burn victim. Would an attendant please call in?"

Jill pressed the button to close the big garage door and got into the passenger seat. She pulled the PCR box out of its holder, took out a fresh prehospital care report, and jotted down the time of the ambulance response and the address and nature of the call. As we sped down Route 10,

she started to fill in the crew members' names, putting
her own name and EMT number in the box marked "In
Charge."

"FPD to 45–01," the voice on the radio said.

Jill keyed the microphone. "Go ahead, FPD."

"Be advised that EMT Williamson will meet you at
the scene."

"10–4," Jill replied.

Good, I thought. Pete Wiliamson is a good EMT. He
worked as a paramedic in the city and was a great person
to have on a bad call, and this one might be a very bad
one. It would be good to have a crew made up entirely of
EMTs. Somehow a call involving severe burns is one of
the most difficult for us to work on. The injuries seem so
devastating, so overwhelming. And, in the bedroom
community of Fairfax, we saw few calls of this type. Pete
would be a great asset.

As the ambulance entered the Floral Court development and turned onto Oak Hill, I saw a teenage boy frantically waving at us. "Please hurry," the boy yelled as we
parked and got out of the rig. "He's in the backyard. He's
burned really bad."

"Go ahead," I yelled. "I'll grab the crash kit and
oxygen." If the burns were to the face, I thought, the
patient could have respiratory problems in addition to
his burns.

With only a moment's hesitation, Jill looked at me,
then turned and hurried toward the backyard, following
the running boy. I grabbed all the equipment I could
carry and ran up behind Jill as she rounded the corner of
the house. A middle-aged man sat awkwardly on a low
stone wall, his body covered with dirt, grass, and leaves.
He was wearing shorts and we could see immediately

that his hands, arms, and legs were badly burned. "Hurry, please," a middle-aged woman next to him pleaded when she saw us approach.

I watched Jill take a deep breath. "Hi, my name is Jill," she said to the man. "What's your name?"

The calm, casual manner that she was trying to project might have seemed forced to Jill, but she was pulling it off. And I was right behind her if she needed me.

"It's Harvey," the man replied through clenched teeth. He was obviously in a great deal of pain.

"Can you tell me what happened?" Jill asked.

"He was pouring starter fluid on the charcoal," the woman said.

Jill turned to the woman. "It's important that he tell me himself," she explained. She needed to determine the patient's level of consciousness, and the best way of doing that was to see if his responses were appropriate.

"The charcoal wouldn't light," he said. "It just needed a bit more juice. It hurts so much."

"I'm Jill, Harvey. Let me examine you. Ed," she said to me, "call in and have them launch the helicopter."

"Don't touch me," Harvey said.

Without touching the burned area, Jill examined her patient, checking his breathing and his vital signs.

"The helicopter is in the air," I told her a few moments later. "They've got an ETA of seven minutes."

"A helicopter?" the woman said. "Is it that serious?"

"It's the best way," Jill said. She looked at me over her shoulder. "Ed, would you get the water gel?"

I sprinted back to the rig and pulled out the orange canister. Water gel consists of sheets of heavy gauzelike fabric impregnated with a gooey substance that both cools the burn and reduces the risk of infection. The sheet in the large canister was big enough to cover the patient's entire body. I also grabbed two packages of smaller ones for wrapping limbs, fingers, and toes.

I ran back to the house. "He's got burns on his hands, both arms, and the front of both legs," Jill said. I could see that Harvey's skin was blackened on his hands and his lower legs. His upper legs and thighs as well as his arms were blistered, with skin sloughing off in some places.

"Oh, God," Harvey said. "It hurts like hell. Can you give me something for the pain?"

"We're not permitted to give any medication," Jill replied, "but this water gel is very cooling. It should make you a bit more comfortable. Then we'll get you to the hospital as quickly as possible. Any trouble breathing?"

"No," he answered, taking an easy, deep breath.

"Good," Jill said. No facial involvement and easy breathing probably meant that the most serious complication, respiratory compromise from smoke or superheated air, probably had been avoided.

"What hurts the most?" Jill asked.

"My arms and thighs," Harvey replied.

Jill was not surprised that the less severely burned areas hurt the most. Harvey's hands and lower legs had been so badly burned that the nerve endings had been destroyed. He could not feel anything in those places.

"FPD to 45–01."

I keyed the mike on my portable radio. "–01."

"Be advised the LZ will be in the open area at the end of Oak Hill. The fire department is on location."

"10–4," I said, aware only now that I was hearing sirens. "We'll be on our way in just a minute."

By now Pete Williamson had arrived on the scene. He went over to Jill. "What do we have?" he asked.

Jill glanced at him as she worked on her patient. "Second- and third-degree burns on his hands, arms, and legs. I'd estimate about 36 percent," she said, recalling the rule of nines. That system allows us to estimate the percentage of the body burned. The head and arms each are counted as one 9, the front and back of the body and each leg are counted as two 9s. The sum of the eleven 9s represents 99 percent of the body surface. The final 1 percent is used for the genitals. Both arms and the front half of each leg added up to four 9s, or 36 percent of the body surface.

"You using water gel?"

"Yes," she said firmly. Many EMTs still used dry, sterile dressings for burns, but Jill had decided to use the gel.

"Okay," Pete said with only a moment's hesitation. "It's messy but let's do it. How about getting him down on a board first?"

I could see Jill considering. "Good idea," she said. "Let's do a standing take-down."

Good job, I thought. She was asserting authority but not reluctant to take suggestions. "Sir," Jill said. "Can you stand?"

Harvey stood up and Jill placed the long backboard behind him. I reached under Harvey's right arm and grabbed one of the board's handholds. Pete did the same thing under Harvey's left arm. Jill moved around in front of her patient. "Just relax, sir. These guys are going to lower you down to the ground. It feels weird, but really they won't drop you."

While Jill spoke, Pete and I slowly lowered the

board, with Harvey against it, to the ground. Then Jill unwrapped the large-size water gel sheet and covered Harvey with it from waist to toes. While she made sure that the goo covered his burns, Pete wrapped his right hand in the smaller wet dressing. I tucked his lesser-burned left hand under the large sheet. "We need to monitor your temperature," Jill said to Harvey. "This stuff can get sort of cold."

Harvey's face relaxed a bit. "Cold would be a blessing," he said.

"Is it helping?" Jill asked.

"Yeah, it really is. Maybe this isn't as bad as I thought."

"Bruce really saved you," the man's wife said. She turned to Jill. "He covered Harvey with a towel and rolled him to put the fire out."

"You're right, ma'am," Jill said. "He probably saved your husband from much worse burns."

"Where is he? Is he burned?" Pete asked.

"I'm here," a voice said. "And I'm fine. Just shaken up a bit."

"I'll go check him out," Pete said, "if that's all right with you, Jill."

"Great," Jill said.

Within ten minutes of our arrival, we had dressed and bandaged Harvey's burns, obtained another set of vitals, and loaded him into the ambulance for the short trip to the helicopter landing zone.

By the time we arrived at the field at the end of Oak Hill, the helicopter was already on the ground. Carrie VanWyk and Sharon Blackstone were waiting for us. "Yuck," Carrie said to the crew, out of the patient's hearing. She looked at Sharon and said softly, "You wouldn't want to crew chief this one, would you? I hate water gel. It's messy and so slippery."

"Not a chance," Sharon said. "This one's all yours."

Jill looked suddenly doubtful. I remembered that she had rejected Pete's suggestion about dry dressings and used the water gel. "Should we have bandaged dry?" Jill asked.

"Nope. This stuff is great for the victim. It's just hell for those of us who have to work with him. But"—she sighed—"he's the most important fellow here. Us poor nurses just have to suffer along." She grinned at Harvey, who almost grinned back.

Jill grinned as well, then filled Carrie in on the patient's condition. In what seemed like only moments, Carrie had a line started, pumping intravenous fluid into Harvey's body to make up for the inevitable fluid loss due to the burns, and Sharon had the helicopter's carry-board ready for Harvey's backboard. As four firefighters from the LZ team carried Harvey toward the chopper, I questioned Carrie. "How is he?"

"He'll live, and with enough morphine, he won't wish he hadn't."

"What will happen to him?" Jill asked. "I've never treated a burn patient before."

"The most important thing is fluid replacement. In the burn unit, they'll carefully try to replace the fluid his body is losing with the exactly correct amount of IV solution," Carrie explained. "Too little and he goes into hypovolemic shock. Too much and the fluid leaks into the tissues and adds to the swelling. They will actually weight him every day to calculate his exact needs."

By now they had Harvey in the helicopter. "He'll eventually be fine," Carrie said as we walked with her toward the chopper. "His hands will present the most difficulty, and he'll have to undergo lots of physical therapy. But you guys acted quickly and correctly. And that friend of his probably saved him from additional months of treatment."

Jill, Pete, and I waved as Carrie climbed into the back of the chopper. As it lifted off, we walked back to the ambulance. "Nice job, Jill," Pete said. "You handled that like an expert."

"You really did," I said.

"Thanks," Jill said. "It was great knowing you two were backing me up."

Over the years since, Jill has become a great crew chief, assertive but able to accept the suggestions of her crew. When I see her in action, I feel good that I was there when she finally learned to trust in her ability.

Chapter 8

This story was told to me by an attending physician in the trauma center.

Glen Markum was nineteen and in his freshman year at the local community college. An outsider all through his high school career, Glen had finally found a group of friends who shared his interest in psychology. The members of the informal psych majors' society were amused at their acronym, PMS. The acronym annoyed the female members of the group, but not enough to induce them to withdraw. The fifteen or so members got together every Friday evening at their table at the Iron Skillet, a restaurant and bar about two blocks away from the edge of the campus.

"Father," one called then took a long swallow of his Sam Adams.

"Mother," several voices yelled.

"Son," another called.

"Daughter."

"Shit," the Sam Adams drinker said.

"On a shingle," one said.

"Damn," Glen said, swallowing the last of the beer in his bottle.

"Defecation," said a third.

"So what's this all supposed to prove?" a slender girl with straight blond hair asked.

"It's just word association," Glen said, glad to have at least a small conversation with Marny Krasner, the blonde, who was new to the group. A friend of Ashley Grady's, Marny had joined them at the Iron Skillet for the second week in a row.

"So what's it good for?"

"It shows up hidden feelings," the Sam Adams drinker said. "It's like if when we say 'father' you say something sexual, we know that you've been sexual with your father."

"Sounds like you're prying into things that are none of your business," Marny said. "And Ashley said you were nice guys." She grinned at her friend, who sat on the other side of Glen. He was delighted at the seating arrangement since whenever the two girls wanted to talk, they had to lean across him.

"Oh, we are nice guys," Glen said. "And you don't have to answer if you don't want to."

"No," a boy with heavy eyebrows and a perpetual scowl said. "We would never pry into your sexual dealings with your father."

"Yeah," a slightly older boy with thick bifocals said, warming to the subject. "What do we care that you and your father fuck like bunnies every night?"

"That's enough, Scap," Glen said. "Watch your language."

"English," Scap said. "Watch yours?" He giggled.

"Okay," the Sam Adams drinker said. "Let's get serious here. The good news is"—he paused for effect, then continued—"I got them."

All eyes at the table turned to stare at him. There were a

few murmurs of "Really," "Right on," and "That's great" around the table.

Marny winked at her friend Ashley. "Got what?" she said with mock innocence.

The Sam Adams drinker reached into his pocket, pulled out an envelope, and emptied the contents, small pieces of blotter paper with an inked initial on one side, into the palm of his hand. "Acid," someone whispered.

"Just for experimental purposes," Sam Adams said, sotto voce. He passed one to each of the group. "We gotta know what it's like."

A few of the members of PMS dropped the bits of paper back into the envelope; others popped the papers into their mouth and washed them down with a swig of beer.

Marny grinned. "I knew he'd get them," she said to Ashley, across Glen's chest. Each of the girls popped a square of paper into her mouth and swallowed. "Come on, Glen," Marny said. "You're going to join us, aren't you?"

Glen had never tried acid before, although several of the group's members had. Usually he managed to palm his paper, then, when everyone stopped noticing anyone's comings and goings, he would slip the paper into his pocket and throw it out later. "Sure I am," he said, popping the paper in his mouth and taking a large swallow of beer.

"You're going to love this," Ashley said, then put another square into his shirt pocket. "For later."

"Fairfax Police to the ambulance. We need you to respond to an intoxicated youth who needs medical attention in the park by the tennis court. You'll see the squad cars."

"10–4," Heather Franks said into the mike. "45–01

will respond to the tennis court for an intoxicated youth."
Grabbing her jacket, Heather, her husband, Tom, and
Sam Middleton trotted into the garage. Sam, that night's
crew chief, and Heather sat in the front and pulled the
orange-and-white ambulance from its bay while Tom
closed the garage doors. When he was safely in the back
of the rig, Sam flipped on the lights and Heather turned
the siren control to wail.

"I thought we didn't do drunks," Heather said.

"We do when the police dispatch us," Sam said over
the alternately rising and falling sound of the siren. "We
have no choice. They call, we haul. That's all." He snick-
ered yet again at the old joke.

"But why do they have to call us?" Tom moaned. "Let
the guy sleep it off."

Sam maneuvered around the cars as they pulled over
ahead of him. "Maybe he's had so much that it's alcohol
poisoning."

"Notice how you two say 'he' all the time," Heather
said. "Drunks aren't always men."

"But they usually are." Sam flipped off the siren as he
pulled the ambulance into the parking lot for the tennis
courts. He saw three black-and-white police cars at the far
end and pulled to a stop beside one of them. Tom grabbed
a crash kit and the three EMTs walked toward a knot of
officers. As Sam made his way between a kneeling Eileen
Flynn and a crouching Chuck Harding, he saw that the
two officers and four civilians were holding a screaming,
struggling boy in his late teens.

"They're coming!" the boy screamed, trying to free
himself from the arms holding him. "They're coming!"
He kicked and almost managed to get one leg free.

Another member of the crowd grabbed his thigh and leaned on it. "Don't let them take me!"

"What's going on?" Sam asked.

Chuck filled him in. "We got a call from a cell phone from one of the tennis players. This kid ran into the court area and began screaming. He threw a few chairs, then curled up in one corner and began to cry. When Chuck arrived, the kid freaked—I guess because of the uniform. I'm not at all sure how we got him down." He handed Sam a small piece of paper. "This was in his pocket."

"Shit," Sam muttered. "Acid."

"That's what we figure. And a bad one."

"AOB?" he asked, wondering about alcohol.

"Some," Eileen said, "but we think this is mostly the acid."

Chuck continued. "We called the trauma center and they said to bring him to the ER. We need you to transport him."

The boy on the ground continued to thrash and moan. "How the hell are we supposed to do that?" Heather muttered.

"We'll get him into a Reeves," Sam said. "He's clearly a danger to himself so we can legally transport him, even if we have to do it in restraints."

Tom and Heather went to one of the side compartments of the ambulance and brought out the Reeves stretcher. They laid it on the ground to one side of the struggling boy. "They're murdering me!" he shrieked. "They're going to kill me! Help me!"

"The best way to transport him," Sam said, "is to get him on this, facedown, with his arms at his sides." Sam pulled each side of the three long straps out from the sides of the Reeves. If the crowd could get the boy on it, they could roll it tightly around him to both keep him from hurting himself and keep him controlled.

Sam knelt beside the boy. "Do we know his name?" he asked.

"No," Eileen said. "We haven't been able to get to his wallet."

"Son," Sam said loudly, hoping the boy could hear and process. "My name's Sam and we're going to take good care of you." His voice, usually gruff and gravelly, was soft and soothing. Unfortunately, it had no effect on the youth, who stared at him uncomprehendingly, his pupils widely dilated.

Heather took over, hoping that a woman's voice might help. "And I'm Heather," she said. "We're here to help you." Her voice had no effect either so she shrugged and looked at Sam. Since they were unable to make meaningful contact with the patient, this transport would have to be done the hard way.

"Okay, guys, I think the best way to do this is to put him on the Reeves faceup, then turn him over. Can we all lift?"

"Ready," a few voices said, readjusting handholds on his legs and arms. The two officers, one on each side, grabbed the boy's belt, and Sam controlled the boy's head to ensure that no injury resulted from moving his still-thrashing patient. Heather and Tom controlled the Reeves and looked to grab any part of the boy's anatomy that slipped from anyone's control.

"All right everyone, let's do this," Sam said. Reasonably efficiently, two cops, three EMTs, and four bystanders managed to get the kicking and screaming young man onto the Reeves. As they turned him over, despite everyone's efforts, the boy managed to free one arm and hit Tom in the face. The still-shrieking boy was quickly subdued, rolled in the Reeves, and strapped tightly inside.

Tom stood up, rubbing his aching jaw. "You okay?" Sam asked.

"Yeah. Just angry at myself for not staying out of the way better."

"What the hell is the hospital going to do with him?" Heather asked as they placed the Reeves on the stretcher and fastened the gurney straps around the boy.

"God only knows," Sam said.

It had been a relatively calm evening in the St. Luke's ER. Julie Gilmore, that evening's attending physician, was just catching up on some overdue paperwork when the radio squawked. "45–01 to St. Luke's ER."

M.J. Kendall, an ER nurse, walked over to the receiver and pressed the button. "St. Luke's on. Go ahead."

"Good evening, St. Luke's," a voice said. There were sounds of yelling in the background. "We're inbound with an approximately twenty-year-old male. We suspect he's ingested a harmful substance. We have no vitals at this time and our ETA is about three minutes." The ER staff had become almost silent, all ears tuned to the unusual transmission.

"What's the patient's chief complaint?" M.J. asked.

The reply was covered with a loud scream. "Say again, 45–01?"

"The patient is currently in a Reeves and is complaining of everything. He's got an altered level of consciousness and is extremely combative."

"Shit," Julie muttered. "Just what we need." She caught M.J.'s eye. "Ask them if we'll need extra security."

"45–01," M.J. said into the mike, "should we summon additional security personnel?"

"That might be wise," the voice from the ambulance said. "There are only three of us."

"10–4. We'll await your arrival."

"With delightful expectation," ER nurse Carol Marks said in her best sarcastic tone.

"I can't wait," M.J. said, replacing the mike in the holder. Then he picked up the phone, dialed the security desk, and requested three additional guards.

During the lull before the storm, they moved two patients out of the observation cubicles into rooms in the rear of the ER. "It'll be quieter there," M.J. told a woman waiting for a plastic surgeon to fix a deep laceration on her forehead. Fortunately for the woman, she had suffered only mild damage in a three-car accident.

"Much quieter," Carol told an eighty-three-year-old man whose difficulty breathing had been almost completely alleviated with high-flow oxygen. He was resting comfortably, and with his pulse-ox reading 98, he could safely be moved out of the direct observation area.

As three uniformed members of the hospital's security force arrived in the ER in response to M.J.'s summons, the bell sounded that announced an ambulance in the bay. Moments later, Sam Middleton walked into the ER and smiled at the group. He approached Julie. "Hi, Doc," Sam said.

"Hi, Sam," Julie said. "I thought I recognized your voice. Having fun?" she asked with a wink.

"Oh, just oodles. The kid's still in the rig, rolled

facedown in a Reeves. The cops found this in his pocket." He handed Julie the small square of paper.

"Got it," Julie said. "Is he of age?"

"Yeah. The cops found his wallet. He's nineteen and we've got his name, address, and date of birth."

"Can you safely bring him in here?"

"Oh, he's quite contained now," Sam said, "but noisy. Extreme paranoia. Keeps screaming that 'they're coming,' whoever *they* are. Then he just screams. He hasn't let up since we first picked him up. Of course I have no idea what to do when you unroll him."

Julie sighed. "Okay. Let's see what we've got."

Sam disappeared out the bay doors, then the ER staff heard the commotion. "Help me! They're killing me!"

EMTs wheeled in a stretcher with the rolled-up Reeves on top. It took all three pairs of hands to keep the rocking stretcher from tipping over. "Where do you want him, Doc?" Sam asked.

"Let's try room 6." Room 6, which was usually used for patients who needed quiet, was one of the only ER rooms with a door that could be closed.

Together the group wheeled the stretcher into the quiet room and transferred the young man to the hospital gurney. "Can you stay and help for a few minutes, folks?" Julie asked the crew.

"Sure," Sam said, "if you need us."

"I'll get you for this! I'll tear you apart!" the boy yelled, his voice hoarse from all his screaming.

The three security guards and the three EMTs positioned themselves around the Reeves. Julie reached down and palpated the boy's head. "No sign of head injury. Did you get to do any survey?" she asked Sam.

"Eyeball only. He was faceup when we got there and

we couldn't really touch him. But I saw no sign of any injury of any kind."

"Good. Well, we've got to unstrap him," Julie said. "M.J.," she said to the nurse, "get me ten milligrams of Valium and bring another ten right behind in case we need it." She turned her attention to the assembled group. "We'll unstrap him and hold him down. I'll check him over as quickly as I can, then we'll get some Valium into him. Maybe we can at least get some vitals and see whether anything else is wrong."

"Whenever you're ready," one of the guards said.

"Let's do it," Julie said.

On a nod from Julie, the six unfastened the straps, unrolled the Reeves, and grabbed for the boy's body. With Heather controlling his head, one guard on each arm, a guard and Tom leaning on his legs, and Sam lying across the boy's midsection, the patient was almost completely immobile. "Son," Heather said. "Calm down. We're trying to help you."

"That's good," Julie said. "He probably can't hear you, but try to get through to him anyway." As Heather attempted to make contact with the boy, Julie ran her trained hands over his body, checking for any sign of injury. Once she had assured herself that the cause of his acute paranoia was the LSD he had injested, she took a pair of blunt-ended trauma shears and cut the sleeve of his shirt. She quickly injected 10 milligrams of Valium into his upper arm. When the thrashing didn't slow in two minutes, she injected a second hypo of Valium. "You guys okay?" she asked the group still holding the struggling boy.

"Help me!" the boy yelled. "They're murdering me!"

"Okay so far," Tom said.

Julie grabbed the boy's wrist but was unable to count his rapid pulse. "I don't think there's anything else wrong, but we'll check him further when he calms." Three minutes later, when the boy was still out of control, Julie gave him 10 more milligrams of Valium. "You know, it's moments like this when I wish I had a video camera."

"How come?" Heather asked.

Julie sighed. "This asshole, pardon my language but I have little sympathy, won't remember what an idiot he was tonight. I would love to be able to show him. Maybe it would keep him from doing this again."

As the boy's struggles slowed a bit, Heather asked, "Will he have flashbacks?"

"He might. The real danger is that LSD can exacerbate any underlying psychological problems a person might have." Since the boy hadn't yet completely calmed, Julie gave him a fourth Valium shot.

As the young man slipped into a stupor, the group members relaxed their grip. Rubbing their arms and the backs of their necks, the three guards returned to their posts. Then together Sam, Heather, and Tom walked out of the small room. "Hey, baby," Heather said to her husband, "you got hit. It's turning wonderful colors." She touched the swelling, reddening area on Tom's cheekbone.

"Shit," Tom said. "I sure felt it when he belted me, but I didn't know he'd gotten me hard enough to leave a mark." He touched his cheek.

Heather quickly grabbed a specially constructed plastic sleeve, filled it with crushed ice from the ice machine, and folded it shut. "Here," she said.

As Julie walked out of the small room, she turned

toward Tom, concerned. "Want me to have a look at that, Tom?"

"Nah," Tom said. "The skin's not broken. He just punched me."

"You sure? No teeth loose?"

Tom moved his jaw around and ran his tongue along the surfaces of his teeth. "I'm okay. Just pissed."

"If you're sure . . . " Julie said.

Tom pressed the ice pack against his swollen cheek. "I'm sure. It's no worse than I get playing volleyball."

"Okay. Just keep the ice on it for a while and if you have any trouble, come see me in the morning. I'm here till noon."

"Will do."

"What's going to happen to that boy now?" Heather asked.

"We got his information so we'll call someone to come and pick him up in the morning. He'll sleep it off and, unfortunately, won't remember anything."

"Then he'll probably do it again."

"Yeah," Julie said. "And we'll see him again too."

In these days of more limited health insurance and more difficult access to the private medical system, many people are forced to use the clinic and emergency room facilities at the trauma center for routine medical care.

Dr. Janine Singh looked down at the chart in her hand, then at the elderly lady sitting on the bench. "I'm so sorry that you've had to wait so long, Mrs. Henderson," the doctor said, taking a seat beside the nicely groomed, gray-haired woman. "We've had a hectic morning." Hectic, she thought. That's an understatement. Two heart

attacks, three patients from a serious motor vehicle accident, in addition to the regular flow of those in need of
urgent care. On days like this, those who could wait got
pushed to the bottom of the stack of charts in the "nonurgent" box. She looked at the chart with its green "this-
one-can-wait" sticker.

The older woman put her paperback novel aside and
patted the doctor's hand. "You look beat, dear. I'm so
sorry to bother you with my little problems."

"It's not little if it's your problem," Dr. Singh said.
"Tell me about your pain."

The woman raised a wrinkled hand and rubbed a spot
in her hair at the back of her skull. "I have a lump and it
hurts a lot. Lumps always frighten me."

"Of course they do, so let me feel it." Dr. Singh
put on a pair of latex gloves, then palpated the hard
bump. "Do you have any other symptoms? Anything
else bothering you?"

"No," the woman said. Then she winced as the doctor
touched the sore spot.

"Generalized headache? Any change in your eating or
bowel habits?"

"No, nothing. Just the lump."

"We can get a scan," she said, then asked, "but have
you by any chance fallen in the past week or so?"

"Why, yes," Mrs. Henderson said, studying Dr. Singh's
face through her thick glasses. "How did you know, dear?"

Dr. Singh couldn't help but smile at the charming
woman. "Tell me about how you fell."

"Oh, it was silly. I slipped on some wet leaves in the
backyard and went flat down on my back. Hit pretty hard
and knocked the wind out of me."

"Any loss of consciousness at the time?"

"No, dear," the woman said. "I just lay there for a few minutes, then got up and went back to my garden."

Dr. Singh ran her trained fingers over the woman's upper spine and head. "Any pain in your neck or skull after that? Any bad headaches, dizziness, vomiting, blurred vision?"

"Oh no, dear. Nothing like that. But I do remember that when I washed my hair the back of my head hurt like crazy. Is that important?"

Dr. Singh turned the woman in her seat so she could see the back of her head. She carefully parted the strands of gray hair and looked at her scalp at the site of the swelling. "Well, Mrs. Henderson, I think that what happened is that when you fell, a small pebble or something like that got under your skin. Then it healed over and now it's just a bit irritated. We can do some X rays to confirm that if you like."

Mrs. Henderson felt the back of her head and smiled. "But of course you're right. That must be what happened." She took a deep breath. "I'm so relieved. I'm sure I don't need any X rays." She leaned closer and almost whispered. "I have no insurance, you see. But should we do anything to get the rock out?"

"I would leave it alone for the moment. I can make an appointment for you at the walk-in clinic in a week or so, but I think that the pain will subside and nothing will really need to be done at all."

"Oh, Doctor, that's just fine. Can I just call the clinic if I need to see someone?"

"Certainly. Any time. And if you feel anything that you're not sure of, come right in."

"Oh, but I will. I only came here because I was a bit

frightened. The doctors in the clinic are really nice, but I wanted someone, you know, more involved."

Dr. Singh made some notes on Mrs. Henderson's chart, then looked at the woman and smiled. "You would have been out of here in half the time if you'd gone to the clinic."

"I know dear," the older woman said, patting Dr. Singh's hand again, "but then I wouldn't have met you."

Often, although a patient demands treatment, what he wants isn't medically necessary. At those times, when it is most difficult to make the patient understand the system, tact and diplomacy are the doctor's most important weapons.

Nunzio Scarlatti and his son Tony arrived at the triage desk at St. Luke's late one afternoon. A painting contractor, Tony still wore his paint-spattered shoes. Nunzio, called Papa by his six children and nineteen granchildren, was dressed in a simple faded work shirt and faded jeans. His arm was in a sling Tony's wife had bought at the local pharmacy.

Once Erika Morely, who was working at the triage desk that day, had gathered the necessary information, Nunzio's chart was placed in the "nonurgent" bin. He and Tony waited for over an hour to be seen.

"I see you have a problem with your elbow," Dr. Bruce Brown said. A third-year resident in emergency medicine, Bruce had dark-brown skin, very close-cropped hair, and a smile that could light up several states. He sat beside the older man on a bench at one end of the emergency room.

"Papa's in a lot of pain," Tony said, leaning across his father. "It's his elbow."

"I'm sorry to hear that, Mr. Scarlatti," Bruce said to the older man.

"He doesn't speak any English," Tony said, his accent thick but clearly understandable. "That's why I took time off from work to come here with him. But he can't stand the pain any longer."

"Yes," Bruce said, reading the summary that Annie had prepared, "I see that. But from what I read here, your father fell a year ago. Why don't you tell me the whole story again?"

"Papa fell a year ago. We were living in Philadephia then and the doctors had to operate. They put some metal pieces inside to hold it together."

While Tony spoke, Bruce pushed the sling to one side and carefully examined the man's elbow. The area from mid-humerus to the elbow was deformed and swollen hard, though not red or hot to the touch. "Okay. Then what?"

"Well, he fell again a few months later. He didn't want to go to the doctor again so he just left it."

"The bone wasn't set the second time?" As they spoke the doctor slowly moved the older man's arm to ascertain the elbow's range of motion. The arm would extend until it was about 15 degrees from straight and would flex only to about 110 degrees. From watching the man's reaction to the motions, Dr. Brown gathered that the movement seemed to cause him discomfort, yet he didn't grimace or make any sound.

"No. He said that the metal pieces would hold it this time too and he didn't want to go back to the doctor."

Bruce looked dubious but didn't pursue the matter

since it was many months past history. "So what brings him here now?"

"The pain," Tony said simply.

"How long has he had this pain?"

"It's been about three months, but it keeps getting worse."

"What brought him in today and not yesterday or last week?" Bruce asked.

Tony spoke to his father, then to Bruce. "He says that he can't stand the pain any more."

The doctor spoke to the older man as Tony translated. "Mr. Scarlatti, where exactly is the pain?" Nunzio pointed to the entire deformed area and his son continued, "He says it all hurts and now he can't move it much at all. He keeps it in the sling and that makes it a little more comfortable."

"Does he take medicine for the pain?"

Tony translated and then answered. "He says no. He doesn't take medicine. He wants to have a room here so they can fix his arm and help his pain."

"Okay," Bruce said, standing and writing on the chart. "Let's get an X ray and see what we can do."

Since the ER was crowded, it was another hour before Bruce was able to look at the X ray with Steve Presley, the senior X-ray tech on duty that afternoon. "Well, the pin's clearly visible," Steve said, running his fingers over the picture. "And there's lots of calcification and bone fragments." He pointed to several areas of white on the X ray's dark background. "You mean he didn't have this second break treated?"

"It seems not," Bruce said. "Let me get Julie in here." As a resident, he could gather information and make tentative diagnoses and treatment plans, but everything had to go through the senior attending physician. "Julie," he called, seeing her in the hall. "Can you look at this a moment?"

Julie joined the two men in the tiny X-ray cubicle. "Distal humerus. That's a nasty break but past. What's the complaint now?"

Bruce related the patient's history succinctly. "He says he's in a lot of pain. There's deformity but no soft swelling, no heat, no redness or extreme point tenderness."

"He'll need to be seen in the ortho clinic," Julie said.

"Yeah, I assumed so. He's not going to be happy. He wants to be admitted."

"Not a chance," Julie said, counting the serious cases backed up in the ER because there were no beds available in the hospital. "This isn't urgent."

"I know that," Bruce said, "and you know that, but convincing him and his son isn't going to be easy."

"Do you want me to see them?" Julie asked.

"No. I'll take care of it. Let me call the ortho clinic and set them up with an appointment. Then I'll try to make them understand."

"Okay," Julie said. "If you need me, just yell."

It was almost half an hour later when Bruce finally had a moment to call the clinic and set Mr. Scarlatti up with an appointment for three days later. He prepared a discharge form, then returned to the bench where the two men waited. "Well, Mr. Scarlatti," he said, "I've made you an appointment with an ortho . . . a bone doctor. He'll see you in the orthopedic clinic on Thursday."

"But what until then?" Tony said, talking to Bruce and translating almost simultaneously.

"He can take medicine for the pain. Tylenol or Advil."

"But can't he stay here?"

"Sir," Bruce said, looking directly at the older man, "this isn't anything new."

Tony kept up a continual translation, and it was clear that Mr. Scarlatti wasn't happy with the doctor's responses. "But he's in terrible pain," the son said. "Can't he stay in a room here? They can fix his arm and the pain too."

"I'm really sorry, sir," Bruce said to Mr. Scarlatti, "but this isn't the kind of thing we keep people here for."

The discussion continued for another five minutes, but in the end, Mr. Scarlatti signed the discharge paperwork and his son took their copy. Bruce pointed to a phone number on the sheet. "I've already made the appointment for you. It's at one o'clock on Thursday. Just call this number the day before and tell them you're coming."

"We come back here?" Tony asked.

"No. Not to this room. The ortho—bone clinic is at the other end of this building. There are big signs." He pointed to where he had written ORTHOPEDIC CLINIC on the paper. "Look for that sign."

"But what about the pain?"

"I suggested here"—Bruce pointed,—"that he take Advil or Tylenol. It's all written out here."

Patients were starting to back up, and Bruce knew he had to return to work. As Tony was about to say something else, the doctor stood up and turned to walk away. Over his shoulder he said, "I'm so sorry but there isn't more I can do. Just give him something for the pain and bring him back. I have several other patients to see, sir," he said softly. "Take your father home."

"But how can I make him understand?" Tony asked, bewildered.

"I'm sure you can do it. Try to convince him to take something for the pain."

"Convince my dad of something," Tony said with a shrug. "Yeah. Right."

About fifteen minutes later Bruce passed by the bench. Tony and his father were still sitting there arguing.

Chapter 9

In EMS, the weather can be one of our worse enemies. The summer's heat and humidity cause an increase in the number of respiratory and heart problems we have to deal with. Also with the nice weather come bee stings and sports injuries, swimming mishaps and heat exhaustion. In addition, warm sunny weather makes "the country" appealing, so city folks flock to our parks and get into all manner of trouble.

Winter is no friend either. Icy or snow-covered roads cause a dramatic increase in motor vehicle accidents. Our ambulances have the best snow tires and some of the most careful and skilled drivers. For icy and snowy weather the Fairfax rigs have a device that spins three-foot sections of chains beneath the driving wheels for added traction. Occasionally we even press the fire department or the highway department into service to tamp and plow our way to a scene. Once we get there, however, sometimes all our creativity is needed to get a patient safely to the ambulance and then to the hospital.

It was one of those mornings when anyone with any brains wanted nothing more than to push the OFF button on the alarm clock, turn over in bed, and pull the covers up to ear level. Unfortunately, Dan Shaw didn't have that luxury. He had to get to work, period. A plumbing contractor, he knew that soon, with the steadily dropping temperatures and strong winds predicted for today, his phone would be ringing off the hook with complaints of frozen pipes. So, when the alarm sounded and the radio clicked on, he yawned and sat up. "The temperature in Fairfax is a balmy twenty-two this morning," the disgustingly cheerful radio DJ said. "The temperature is dropping steadily and there's a layer of fresh snow over the freezing rain that fell last evening. Be careful out there, everyone. It's slippery as Teflon. If you can, stay home."

"Thanks," Dan muttered.

"And for all you school kids and teachers out there, you can go back to sleep. All the local area schools are closed. We'll have the complete detailed list on the half hour."

"Umm." Jane Shaw moaned. "Great. Good news, I don't have to go to work. Bad news, the kids are home. Will you let them know so I can get a few more minutes down time?"

"Sure, hon." His wife taught third grade at George Washington Elementary, the same school and grade that their younger son, Brian, attended. The older one, Jeff, was in fifth.

After telling the boys that school was closed, Dan showered and dressed in his warmest work clothes, with an extra hooded sweatshirt in case any job was outside. He toasted two Pop-Tarts and, munching, headed for the garage. When he opened the garage door, he squinted outside at the blazing whiteness that assaulted him. The trees were covered with a coating of ice and the long, steeply sloping driveway was a sea of snow. There was a brisk wind, but the three inches of snow wasn't drifting. With a sigh, he knew he'd have to shovel and salt at least the first ten feet, the flat part, so that the car would have some traction making the turn out of the garage. He wouldn't even try to shovel the long hill. He'd just blast through and wait for the snow and ice to melt.

He pulled on his gloves and grabbed the shovel. After one step out of the garage, he realized how right the guy on the radio had been. Beneath the snow lay a thick layer of ice, and the combination was slippery as hell. He put a ten-pound bag of Halite beside the garage door, then closed it behind him to conserve heat. Being careful of his footing, Dan began to shovel.

He had cleared about half of the upper part of the driveway when a bright-red cardinal flew by. As he turned to get a better look, Dan's feet went out from under him and he crashed to the pavement. Although he was able to get his arm out to break his fall, he hit the shovel hard on his right side, which knocked the wind out of him.

As he caught his breath, he knew that, despite the padding provided by his clothes, he had done something to his hip and his wrist. And his right ribs hurt when he tried to take a deep breath. "Shit," he muttered. "I'm in real trouble. Help," he yelled as loudly as he could, his breath making long plumes in the freezing air. "Help me!" He gazed at the closed garage door, then at the front door, both so far away. "Help." He slumped, feeling totally defeated.

In preparation for standing or crawling, Dan tried to turn onto his side. Shafts of pain stabbed through him from both his side and his hip. Breathless, he rolled onto his back again. He'd have to get help, but how could he drag himself to a door and get inside? Since the front door was fifty feet away and up seven steps, he decided to try for the garage, which was closer. At least, he thought, even if I can't open the damn door, maybe there will be some heat coming from under it. Sweating from the exertion, it took about ten minutes for him to slide to the garage, but he couldn't figure out how to get the door open. Feeling thoroughly defeated and in considerable pain, he slumped against the wooden door frame and rested.

As he lay still and caught his breath, he started to shiver uncontrollably, which made his ribs hurt. He banged on the garage door but got no response. After about fifteen minutes of pounding, Dan dimly heard his two boys bound out the front door.

"Hey, Dad," Jeff asked as they rounded the corner of the house and saw him, "are you okay?"

"Get Mommy," he said, his words slurred. "Fast."

The boys dashed into the house and, almost immediately, Jane appeared in Dan's field of vision. "What happened?" she said. "Are you okay?"

"No. I fell." His words were punctuated by bouts of full-body quaking shivers and quick shallow breaths. "I'm hurt. So cold. Get help."

He watched Jane turn and say to the boys, "Get the blankets off your beds and cover your father. I'm calling 911."

Every year my condo association hires a wonderful landscaping and outdoor maintenance contractor. By the time I got up that morning, my nice flat parking area was plowed, shoveled, and salted. I dressed and started my car, allowing it to run for a few minutes so the covering of ice would be melted from the windows. Then I had errands to run.

The first ambulance was out for a person who had collapsed while shoveling snow. Heart attacks are not unusual on snowy mornings.

"Fairfax Police to the ambulance. A second crew is needed for a man who fell in his driveway. The address is 789 Hunter's Hill Road. Be advised it's a long driveway just after the SLOW CURVE sign."

I waited, hoping someone else would call in, but when the second page sounded, the dispatcher said he still needed a full crew. Although I'm a confirmed couch potato and I hate winter, snow, ice, cold, and everything that goes with them, I called in.

"Pete Williamson just called in. He's picking up the rig, Joan," Mark Thomas told me.

"Okay," I said. "I'll respond to the scene."

As I drove at thirty miles per hour up the parkway, I realized that this could be a difficult transport. Although the parkway was plowed and sanded, the entrance and exit ramps were still covered with ice and the side roads were a disaster. I turned onto Hunter's Hill Road, found the curve sign, and saw that the rig was parked just far enough into the driveway that it didn't impede traffic. I drove farther down the road, parked in a small pull-off, and walked carefully back to the driveway. As I looked up, the task of me getting up, then us getting our patient down the driveway seemed daunting. The driveway was almost fifty feet long and steeply sloped to a flat area at the top.

I saw fresh footprints off the side of the driveway and followed them up, stepping on what turned out to be snow-covered grass rather than pavement. At the top I found our patient under the care of Pete Williamson and Phil Ortiz. The man, who was shivering violently, was covered with blankets.

"Hi, Joan," Pete said. "This is Dan and he took a bad fall. He's got a probable broken right wrist and maybe a rib or two. He's also got severe pain in his right hip, and I think he's mildly hypothermic."

Phil looked up from the gauge on the BP cuff. "BP 125 over 76," he said. "Pulse 60 and respirations 24 and shallow. He says it hurts to take a deep breath but his lung sounds are normal."

"What do you need," I asked, "and, more important, how are we going to get him down this driveway?"

Pete sighed. "We need to splint his wrist. The rest, I don't know yet."

I heard a siren and looked puzzled.

"I called for the fire department rescue truck," Pete said. "I thought we might need muscle, and someone may have a bright idea about how to get the rig up here or get him down there. Bring a splint, straps, and a long-board for starters."

"Will you need collars and such?"

"I don't think so. He says he hit on his side and arm, and he was well padded with several layers of clothing. There's no head, neck, or back pain and, since I don't want to remove any clothing just yet, I think we can take the chance."

"Okay." As I tramped back to the rig using the already-made path through the grass, I saw several fire-fighters get out of the rescue. I had worked with all these men on numerous occasions.

"Hi, Joan," Ken Stavitsky said. "What have you got?"

"We've got a man who fell, broke his wrist." I pointed up the driveway. "Up there."

"Oh." Ken turned to Mike DeVito. "Let's get some ropes so we can make handholds if we need to."

I found a splint for the man's wrist and a longboard and straps. I also grabbed two chemical heat packs and stuffed them in my jacket pockets. Ken helped me carry equipment back up the hill. We quickly immobilized the man's wrist and carefully logrolled him onto the long backboard. I broke the inside container on the heat packs and allowed the chemicals to mix. Then I put one on either side of Dan's chest, inside his zip-front sweatshirt, and refastened all his clothing.

"I've got an idea on how to get this guy down the driveway," Pete said. "I hate to ask you to make another trip, but I think the Reeves would work."

"I'll go," Phil said.

"Work how?" I asked.

"You'll see," he replied.

Grateful that he had thought of a way to move the patient, I talked with Pete and the injured man until Phil returned with the slatted stretcher. "Are we going to carry him all the way down?" I asked.

"I've actually got a better idea," Pete said. "We're going to make a toboggan."

"A *what*?" Dan asked. "You're going to *slide* me down the driveway?"

"In a way," Pete said. Rather than explaining, he just gave instructions. "Ken, rig a long rope up the driveway and around that tree. And bring me a shorter piece of rope." He indicated a tree about five feet from where we were working. As Ken left to follow instructions, Mike DeVito, Phil, Pete, and I lifted Dan's backboard onto the

Reeves. When Ken handed Pete the end of the rope, now looped around a large pine tree, Pete tied it to the upper handles of the Reeves.

"Okay," Pete explained, "just play out the rope and we'll slowly slide this makeshift toboggan down the driveway." He tied the center of the shorter piece of rope to the handles at the foot end of the Reeves, then crossed to the snow-covered grass on the far side. "This will help keep the sled in the center of the driveway."

"Nice idea," I said, impressed by Pete's ingenuity. Then he and I walked on either side of the ice-covered driveway, guiding the toboggan down the center of the slippery pavement.

It worked amazingly well. In only a few minutes, Dan, on his backboard-Reeves sled, arrived at the foot of the driveway.

From there it was easy. We loaded our now-slightly-warmer patient into the rig and slowly drove him to Fairfax General Hospital.

Three hours later I arrived back at the hospital with the victim of a one-car PIAA. "How's the patient we brought in this morning?" I asked.

"He's warm now, and lucky he didn't get much colder," Dr. Morrison said. "His core temperature was ninety-one when you got him here. He's got two broken ribs and a Colles fracture of the wrist. His hip was badly bruised but nothing was broken. We'll probably keep him overnight just to be sure his lungs are okay and so we can keep him on good strong pain meds. He'll be home tomorrow."

"I guess that's good. If he'd slid all the way down that crazy driveway . . ."

"I heard. That was a neat way you guys got him down."

"All Pete's idea," I said. "I'm so glad he was there. All I could think of was carrying the poor guy down the hill. The bouncing would have been really painful."

"Tell Pete he did really good, will you?"

"Sure will," I said. Boy, do I like having Pete around.

"God, it is really hot," Craig Thomas said to his friend Doug. "I could sure use a Coke."

"Yeah, me too." Fourteen-year-old Doug Johnson wiped his brow and then rubbed his sweaty palms on his Chicago Bulls T-shirt.

"Let's use the soda machine in front of the gas station," Craig said. "Scoop showed me how to get two sodas but only pay for one." Their friend Scoop earned his nickname by always scooping up anything he could get for nothing.

"Yeah? Can we do that?"

"Sure. It's easy. I'll show you." The two boys walked rapidly toward the gas station in the center of Fairfax. When they arrived, they saw that the pumps and the convenience store were sufficiently busy to keep the attendants occupied. "Okay," Craig said. "I'll put the money in. As the machine cycles, put your hand up inside. There's some little doo-hingy that opens, and you can get the next soda in the stack while the first one drops."

"Okay." Doug pushed the plastic door up and, while Craig dropped the proper change into the machine, he reached up inside. As the machinery cycled and Craig's Coke dropped against his forearm, Doug did feel something shift, then he felt his hand get pinched inside the dispenser. "Hey, man, I can't get my hand out. Gimme a yank."

Craig pulled on Doug's arm but nothing gave. He was stuck tightly. "Get me outta here," Doug yelled. "This hurts."

"Well, pull, you jerk."

"I am pulling but my hand won't come out."

"I don't know what you did. When I did it, my hand came right out, and with a soda too." Craig reached in and around Doug's arm and tried to get his Coke. "Hey, with your arm jammed in there I can't get my can out either. I guess I better tell someone."

"Not yet." Doug wiggled and twisted his arm but, although it got increasingly sore, it wouldn't budge. "Okay, I guess you better tell someone," he finally agreed.

I was on duty that afternoon when we were contacted by phone for a standby.

"FVAC, Linda Potemski speaking."

"Hi, Linda. It's Mark Thomas at FPD. The fire department's on the way to the front of the A-Plus minimart in town for a child with his hand stuck in the Coke machine. We just want you to stand by in case he needs attention when they get him out."

Linda looked at me and shrugged. "Okay. 45–01 will be responding to the minimart." She hung up.

Fred Stevens, who has a tendency to "speak his mind," climbed into the driver's seat. We pulled out of the garage and proceeded to the center of town, code 2. "God damn kids," Fred mumbled. "I can't wait until they're back at school."

"Down, Fred," Linda said. "You have no idea what's going on."

"Can't be anything on the up and up if the kid got his hand stuck inside a Coke machine."

Linda and I laughed but quietly we agreed with Fred.

We arrived at the gas station minimart and saw the gathered crowd. We got out and found Police Officer Eileen Flynn standing about ten feet from the machine. With half a dozen firemen gathered around him, we couldn't even see the boy.

"This kid stuck his hand inside the machine trying to get a free Coke," she told us. "When the machine gave the other kid the soda he had paid for, our young Mr. Brilliant got his arm stuck inside."

"Let's try some soap," a voice said.

"We've got someone coming with the key," another said.

"Maybe if the swelling in his hand gets a chance to go down, it will come out," a third said.

"We can use the jaws . . ."

Eileen leaned close to the three of us. "The kid's father is on the way. I reached him at work, and he didn't sound like a happy camper."

I shrugged and, with Linda and Fred, stood aside and let the fire department experts try to extricate the boy's hand. After ten minutes, the boy's arm was still stuck fast.

A panel truck with A&G DISTRIBUTORS on the side pulled up, and a middle-aged man in a delivery uniform got out. "Let me through," he said. "I've got the key to the machine." He inserted the key in the side of the soda machine and tried to open the front panel. With the boy's arm wedged in the opening where the cans come out, the door would open only about three inches.

"We can take the door off the hinges," someone said.

"Yeah, but what good would that do? We can't open the door with this kid's arm in the way."

"Doug Johnson, I'm going to kill you!" a voice boomed. Then a car door slammed.

"That must be the father," Linda said as we watched a middle-aged man in a short-sleeved denim work shirt, jeans, and work boots walk from a pickup truck toward the crowd.

"Dad," the boy yelled. "I'm sorry."

"You're going to be very, very sorry," the man bellowed. He stormed through the group of firemen, reared back, and slammed his fist toward the boy, hitting the soda machine as his son dodged. "Shit," he yelled, shaking his hand, then cuffing the boy hard with his other hand. "I think I broke my fuckin' hand."

Doug suddenly stood up from the crouch he had been forced to maintain while his hand was locked in the soda machine. "I'm unstuck. Hey, I'm unstuck."

"You may be unstuck, but I think you broke my fuckin' hand," the man said to his son, cradling his right fist against his chest with his other arm.

The boy stayed out of arm's reach as the man bellowed.

"Sir," I said, walking up to the father, "why don't you let me check your hand?" Linda walked up to the boy and said almost the exact same thing. We examined both victims. While Doug was uninjured, we transported his father to FGH, where X rays indicated he had broken two small bones in the palm of his hand.

"Fairfax Police to the ambulance. The ambulance is needed on Hunter's Hill Road near Deerfield for a PIAA."

"10–4," Dave Hancock said. He, Fred Stevens, and I were riding the afternoon shift that Tuesday. "That's a bad stretch. How many serious ones have we had there, I wonder."

With Dave driving, me riding shotgun, and Fred in the back, we pulled out of the garage and onto Route 10 toward the parkway and Hunter's Hill Road. As we approached the accident scene, we saw a line of flares and then a car resting nose-first against a tree. We pulled in behind the wreck, leaving our lights flashing to warn other drivers about the accident. I jumped out and walked up to the driver's side of the car. The door was open and an older man was sitting in the car, his feet on the pavement and his head leaning against the headrest.

I looked at the front of the car. There seemed to be no damage at all. The windshield was intact and there were a few papers still on the passenger seat that should have slipped to the floor on impact. "Sir," I said to the driver, "what happened?" The man didn't seem to realize I was speaking. He just continued to gaze straight ahead. "Sir," I said again, "can you speak to me?"

Officer Stan Poritsky walked up behind me. "We found him like this and he hasn't said anything at all. Just stares. I thought he might have a head injury. We've got his wallet." I heard Stan give Fred the man's name, address, and date of birth for our paperwork. "He's seventy-six," Stan said.

I inhaled, wondering about alcohol, but I smelled nothing. "Sir, were you in an accident?" I got no answer from our patient.

Dave had gotten into the backseat of the car and was holding the man's head against the headrest to prevent any additional neck injury. "He's cold," Dave said, "and he's very sweaty." I quickly surveyed the man's body but saw no sign of trauma. After taking a second careful look at his head, I ran my hands over his scalp and neck, checking for lumps, depressions, cuts, or bruises. Nothing.

"Joan," Dave said. "Maybe the disorientation caused the accident, not the other way around."

"I was beginning to think that too, Dave." I took the man's wrist to check his pulse and noticed a medical alert bracelet. I looked at the back of the engraved plate. "We're right," I said. "He's a diabetic and probably is in insulin shock." If he took his insulin in the morning but didn't eat enough breakfast, his blood sugar would fall too low for his body to tolerate. When he was no longer able to manage the car, he either pulled his car over or slowly drove off the road and bumped into the tree.

Fred handed me a cervical collar as a precaution, but as I tried to fasten it, the man became combative. He pushed me away and tried to pull Dave's hand from his head.

"Leave me alone," he cried, his speech a bit slurred.

"Dave," I said, "I think we can risk transporting without immobilizing him. There's no reason to suspect a spinal injury."

"I agree," Dave said, removing his hand from the man's head. "Fighting with him probably will do more harm than good anyway." When the restraint was gone, the man calmed again. Dave took vitals. "BP's 140 over 84, his pulse is 88 and pounding." The man had begun to sweat more profusely, soaking his long-sleeved shirt.

Fred brought the stretcher and we transferred the man to it. We lifted him, sitting up, into the rig and, with Fred driving, headed for the hospital.

"Let's try some glucose," I said. If he was indeed in insulin shock, as I suspected, the sugar would improve his condition quickly and could not do any harm.

Dave fetched the tube of the pink sugary goo we carry, twisted off the top, and squeezed some into our patient's mouth. Although quite a bit drooled out, he swallowed some. Dave squeezed more and he swallowed again. Within five minutes, the tube was empty and the man's condition had begun to improve. I rechecked his pulse and breathing, then put an oxygen mask over his face. About three minutes from FGH I pressed the keys that would open their radio. "45–01 to Fairfax emergency."

"Go ahead, 45–01."

"We are en route to your location with a seventy-six-year-old man who is severely disoriented. Although he was involved in a PIAA, I think his problem is diabetic. He's wearing an ID bracelet and his condition seems to be improving with the glucose we are giving him by mouth. His vitals are BP 140 over 84, pulse was 88 and is now 78, respirations 24, down from 28. Our ETA is about two minutes."

"10–4, 45–01. We'll give you a room assignment on arrival."

"10–4. 45–01 is clear."

By the time we arrived at the hospital, our patient was feeling quite a bit better. He was talking with the nurses by the time we finished our paperwork.

"Glad we found that bracelet," I said as we walked the stretcher back to the rig. "It certainly helped us decide how to treat him."

"Yeah," Dave said. "When we got there I was sure that his problem was related to the accident."

"Me too," Fred said. "Occasionally when you hear hoofbeats, it isn't horses. It really is zebras."

Isabel and Brad Lamont had rejoiced when Isabel finally became pregnant after almost three years of trying. "Not that the attempts weren't fun," Brad told their friends at a celebratory party held when Isabel was entering her fourth month, "but I do prefer to have sex when we want to, not when the thermometer says so."

At her five-month checkup, her obstetrician, Dr. Ciner, did a sonogram and blood tests, then told her that everything was going well. Then the nurse began to tell her about the local hospital's natural childbirth courses and maternity orientation tours. At Isabel's request, Dr. Ciner didn't tell her the sex of her child.

Toward the end of her fifth month, Brad, a computer wizard with a large accounting firm, came to her with bad news. "I'm going to be on an assignment in Seattle for about two months," Brad told her. "It's a short-term thing and the project will be done well before your due date, and, of course, I'll be home on weekends."

"Are you sure it's only for two months? The last two-month assignment lasted seven. I really don't want to have this baby alone."

"You didn't make this baby alone and you won't have him or her alone either. And there's good news too. I got a guarantee that I'll have at least a year here or in the city after the baby's born. No out-of-town stuff." Resigned to their weekday separation, Isabel and Brad made a special effort to enjoy their weekends together.

About 4:15 A.M. one Monday, during Brad's third

week away, Isabel was awakened by a mild lower abdominal pain. Although the pain wasn't rhythmic, it was sufficiently unusual that she called her obstetrician's service. When Dr. Ciner returned her call, he asked, "Any bleeding, fluid flow, anything unusual other than the abdominal discomfort?"

"No."

"Then just sit tight. I'm sure it's nothing. But if anything changes or you're in any way uneasy, call me back." He gave her his home phone number.

About an hour later, the pain became more focused and Isabel became more upset. She called her obstetrician again. "Maybe you'd better get over to the emergency room," he suggested. "Let the doctor in the ER examine you and he'll contact me. I'll call and alert them that you're coming."

"But Brad's not here. He's in Seattle. I don't want to do this alone."

"Can you call some family member, a friend, or a neighbor?"

"There's really no one here for me." Isabel didn't feel close to anyone in Fairfax.

"Then dial 911 and the ambulance will pick you up. I certainly don't want you driving. And tell them, if possible, to take you to the medical center. I'll contact the police, and I can meet you at either FGH or St. Luke's if necessary."

"Okay. I'll call them." As she hung up, she felt another pain deep in her pelvis. These aren't too much worse than menstrual cramps, she thought. I can handle it. It's probably nothing. She dialed 911.

I was riding my usual Sunday midnight shift from home without Ed, who was down with the flu and was sleeping at his house. When the phone rang I cursed. We never get calls on Monday mornings. It had been several months since we'd had to get up in the middle of the night. Now, the one night that Ed didn't ride . . .

"Yeah," I said into the phone. "What have we got?"

"We have a call for a woman in labor at 243 Spring Hill Road. It's the fourth house on the left. Nick Abrams is picking up the rig and Jack McCaffrey will meet you at the scene."

"I'm on my way," I said, already partly dressed. It took only a few moments after I hung up to finish dressing, grab my car keys, and sprint from the house. Woman in labor. Great kind of call, I thought. Maybe I'll get to deliver a third baby.

I drove to Spring Hill Road and, as I turned left, I saw a police car at the top of a short driveway. I pulled in, parked, and walked to the front door. "Ambulance," I called.

"In here." I recognized Merve Berkowitz's voice. I entered the kitchen and found a nice-looking woman dressed in a pair of maternity jeans and a sweatshirt, sitting on a kitchen chair, her head in her hands. It amused me to see how quickly Merve backed away and let me take over.

"Hello. I'm Joan and the ambulance will be here soon."

The woman lifted her head and I saw tearstains on her cheeks. I squatted beside her and put my arm around her shoulders. Unprepared for the misery I saw on her face, I glanced at her belly, not nearly as large as I expect the usual full-term pregnancy to be. "Can you tell me your name?"

"Isabel Lamont. I'm so scared. I'm only just starting my seventh month."

"It's all right. We're here now." I heard the siren. "That's the ambulance. We're going to take good care of both you and your baby."

"My husband flew out early this evening. To Seattle. I thought about calling him but what good can he do from so far away? It'll just scare him." She began to cry again.

"Isabel, look at me," I said, using my most professional-sounding tone. "We are going to get through this. You and I. We're going to get you to the hospital so, if it's really labor, you can deliver a baby. Is it a boy or a girl?"

"Brad, that's my husband, and I didn't want to know until it was born."

"Okay. Let's call the baby Munchkin. 'It' sounds so impersonal. Tell me about the pains."

"I've been checking the clock." She wiped her nose. "They're not too regular and not too bad."

"Okay. That's good. Exactly how far along are you?"

"About twenty-five weeks."

"Is this your first?"

"Yes." She sniffled. "We tried for a long time."

"Well, congratulations. Has your water broken?"

Isabel looked miserable. "About ten minutes ago. I had just gotten dressed and now I'm soaked. I called the doctor and told him."

When she started to cry again I held her tightly. "We'll handle what we have to handle," I said as Nick and Jack arrived with the stretcher. "These are the rest of my crew, Nick Abrams and Jack McCaffrey. Both these guys have kids and I have two myself. We'll take good care of you, I promise."

We spread the sheets on the stretcher and I handed Isabel a blanket. "Isabel, drape this around you and take off your jeans and underpants. If Munchkin decides to be born, those clothes will get in our way just a bit." I winked and, as I held the blanket and assisted her, Isabel removed the clothing from the lower half of her body. We then settled her on the stretcher. "How long have you been having these contractions?"

"About three hours," she said.

"And how long do they last? Have you timed them?"

"Yes. They last just under a minute." She grimaced.

"Are you having one now?"

"Yes," she said.

I jotted the time down on the edge of the report form. "Okay, just try not to tighten up. Breathe in quick, panting breaths. Tell me when the contraction eases. Have you had any childbirth classes?"

The contraction wasn't severe enough to keep her from talking. "No. It was too soon."

"Any desire to push, like you were moving your bowels?"

"No."

"Good. That means nothing's going to happen too soon." I really didn't want to deliver a premature baby.

"It's easing now," she told me.

"Okay." I nodded to Jack and Nick. "Let's go and I'll examine Isabel in the rig."

"Oh," Isabel said as we wheeled her out the front door. "My doctor said I should ask if you can take me to the medical center."

"You mean St. Luke's? Sure." I knew that if she was going to deliver a six-month baby, the hospital's neonatal unit was the best place for her to be.

"The doctor said he'd call the police and find out where you were taking me."

I turned to Merve who nodded. "I'll call headquarters," Merve said, "and tell them to contact your doctor. What's his name?"

"Ciner. David Ciner." She gave Merve the phone number.

"Sure thing. And you're in great hands," Merve said. "They'll take really good care of you."

"Thanks," Isabel said as we lifted her into the rig.

Inside the ambulance, as Nick rounded the rig to the driver's seat, I pulled the blanket aside as another contraction overtook our patient. I opened the OB kit and removed the sterile drapes, quickly placing them beneath Isabel's bottom, around her thighs, and across her abdomen. Then I checked to see whether the baby's head was visible and saw no bulging of the tissues. "No sign of crowning just yet," I said, noting the time of the most recent contraction on my report. "Those last two were about three minutes apart." As Nick backed out of the driveway I took a quick set of vitals. "Everything's looking good," I said.

"I'm so scared," Isabel said. "Can I hold your hand?"

"Of course," I said, taking the woman's sweaty hand in mine. "Tell me about your husband. What does he do that keeps him out of town?"

As we drove down the parkway toward St. Luke's, we talked about anything we could think of, just trying to get through the trip. The contractions were coming regularly at about three minutes apart and I just tried to keep Isabel calm. I checked each time for crowning, but thankfully saw none. When we were about five minutes from the hospital, I called in.

After I had told them the patient's condition, the nurse asked, "Is this Dr. Ciner's patient?"

"Yes, it is."

"Okay. He's here waiting for you."

"That's great," Isabel said as another contraction washed over her.

"Any evidence of crowning?" the voice from the hospital asked.

I had checked with each previous contraction, but she was having another one so I wanted to give them the most updated information. I handed the phone to Jack who said, "We'll let you know in a moment."

I checked and suddenly, at the peak of the contraction, I saw the top of a head appear between the separating tissues. "I see something," I said. "We might have to deliver this baby after all." Terrified, I tried to sound as calm as I could. I remembered from the chapter on childbirth in the EMT textbook that small babies could be born very quickly, with very little discomfort. "I've delivered two others. This might be my third."

While I opened the OB kit, Jack told the hospital what was happening and gave an ETA of five minutes. "10–4. St. Luke's clear," the voice said.

Jack replaced the phone in its cradle and moved to the bench beside me. "Isabel," I said, "you have a choice. Both Jack and I are trained in delivering babies, so you can have me either hold your hand or catch Munchkin. Which would you like?"

She looked at me, then said, "I'll hold Jack's hand. But the baby can't be coming yet. The contractions aren't too bad."

"Well, I don't know about the contractions, but from what I can tell, Munchkin might be ready to see Mommy."

I was terrified. Delivering healthy, full-term babies is really very easy. When I teach the childbirth classes to future EMTs, I tease that you could do it with a catcher's mitt. The mother actually does all the work and you get all the glory. A premature baby is another matter entirely. So much can go wrong. But I couldn't burden Isabel with my fears. I had to appear confident and in charge.

I pulled on the sterile gloves from the kit and, as the rig sped off the exit ramp toward the hospital, I watched as the baby's head appeared. I cradled the tiny head as the shoulders slipped from Isabel's body in a gush of fluid. Be breathing, Munchkin, I prayed silently. As the incredibly slippery hips and legs slid out, the baby gave a tiny, weak cry. I quickly dried Munchkin off as we pulled into the emergency bay at the trauma center.

"It's a girl, Isabel. She's very tiny, but she's breathing on her own."

"Thank God," Isabel said.

I wrapped the infant in a clean, dry towel and laid her on Isabel's belly, arranging a blanket over them both. Then I fastened a barrettelike plastic clamp around the umbilical cord about six inches from the baby and another a hand-span from it. Then I cut the cord between the clamps.

The back doors of the ambulance opened and several gowned and masked figures appeared. "Delivered?" one asked.

"Yes," I said, carefully picking up the newborn.

"That's great. Congratulations, Mom. We've got an isolette right here," one gowned woman said, and I gladly placed the tiny girl in her outstretched hands.

"Has the placenta been delivered?" someone asked me.

"Not yet. The baby only delivered about thirty seconds before we pulled in."

"Okay. If you want," another woman said, "take a moment to get Mom cleaned up and then you can take her upstairs. Dr. Ciner is right here."

Isabel grabbed my arm. "Joan," she said, "could you stay with me? I feel so alone and I'm so scared about the baby. She's so little and so early."

I looked at my watch. 6:15. I had gone off duty at 6:00. I could get a taxi back to my car. I did want to stay with Isabel and see how the baby made out. "Sure. I'll stay with you for a while and get a ride home later. Give me about fifteen minutes to write my report and I'll meet you upstairs." Jack, Nick, and I got Isabel cleaned up and blanketed, and, while the two men wheeled her up to labor and delivery, I wrote the paperwork.

Almost half an hour after the baby girl's birth, I found my way upstairs. Isabel was just being wheeled out of the birthing suite with Dr. Ciner beside her. "Well, hello there," he said to me. "You did just fine. I delivered the placenta but everything you did was just great."

"Thanks. How are you feeling, Isabel?" I asked.

"I'm okay, but I'm wondering about Munchkin." She smiled. "I think I'll call her that until Brad and I can pick a name. They say I can go over to the neonatal area and see her in about an hour. Can you stay till then?"

"Try to kick me out," I said.

As they wheeled Isabel toward her room, I asked the doctor, "Why was the baby born so early?"

"With most neonates we never really know why labor starts early. At her last checkup Isabel was in great shape."

An hour later, with Isabel settled into a wheelchair, we

went over to the neonatal area and found Dr. Leonard Campbell, the neonatalogist in charge of little Ms. Munchkin Lamont. "It's nice to meet you," Dr. Campbell said to Isabel. "You're the mom, but who's this?" he asked, indicating me.

"She's my friend Joan," Isabel said. "She's the one who was in the ambulance and delivered my baby."

"Well, you delivered a fine, small but amazingly healthy baby girl," Dr. Campbell said. "Do you have a name for her?"

"We'll call her Munchkin until my husband gets here. We weren't really ready for this yet."

"Okay. Munchkin is about 1,300 grams—that's not quite three pounds." He turned to Isabel. "I won't give you any details about her condition until we're alone. That's hospital policy. But I can tell you that there isn't anything to worry about right now. We'll have our ups and downs together and she's not out of the woods yet, but I have no reason to expect that your daughter won't get along fine."

"How long will she be here?" Isabel asked.

"I can't tell you definitely because there are a lot of variables, but, as a rule of thumb, babies like Munchkin usually go home sometime around the date they would have been born." He walked us to the large picture window and indicated an area in which the tiny baby lay, surrounded by three gowned, gloved, and masked women.

"Those are your baby's nurses and they've got a few things to do now since she's so new."

"What are all those machines?" Isabel asked.

"They're monitoring every part of your baby. We constantly check her blood pressure, her pulse and respirations and how well her blood is transferring oxygen to all of her body. That way we can give her just the right amount of supplementary oxygen. You'll get used to the equipment quickly and you'll soon learn what each piece does."

"My baby's getting oxygen?"

"Yes. One of the most difficult problems with tiny ones like yours is that their lungs aren't fully developed yet. So we help them breathe."

As we watched, the baby flailed one arm. "She's moving," Isabel said with wonder, tears filling her eyes.

"Sure she is," Dr. Campbell said. "She's a person. She'll cry, eat, and wiggle just like you'd expect. Give us a few hours to get organized and you can even hold her."

"Oh, yes," Isabel said. "That will be great." Together, smiling, Isabel and I left the window.

"You sure seem to have made a beautiful baby," I said.

"And you caught her for me. Thanks."

"You're so welcome. I was glad to be a part of all of this." And poor Ed, I thought. What a night for you to have the flu. You would have enjoyed this so much. You'll be so jealous. And he was.

Chapter 10

EMTs and paramedics deal with pain, fear, and death in many ways. We all face the same problem: how to remain sane, healthy, well-functioning human beings after years of responding to people who are sick, injured, and sometimes dying. How do you continue to feel good about yourself when the life of a twelve-year-old girl slips through your hands despite all of your efforts to keep her alive?

Some of us do it with bravado and arrogance. Some with humor. And some of us cry a lot. Some of us remain the same people we were, and some are profoundly changed by our experiences. I have known EMTs and paramedics who start out motivated by a desire to help people and who, after a period of time, become hard, uncaring, and sometimes even cruel to their patients. They will tell you that this is the only way to cope with the daily stress of their job. I have known others, however, who begin as young, arrogant thrill-seekers who care little about people but who grow and mature into warm, supportive professionals able to provide not only physical but also emotional care in a medical emergency.

It was a beautiful Saturday in July. Joan was away for the day so I decided to take my laptop computer to

Fairfax headquarters and work there. The building was usually quiet on beautiful weekend afternoons so I could get some work done without interruption. No phones. No teenage kids. And I was in the mood to take whatever calls came in.

As I worked in the office at the back of the building, I heard the TV in the crew room. Someone else was hanging out, waiting for a call.

The tones went off and, through the building-wide PA system, I heard the familiar voices of police dispatcher Mark Thomas and Nick Abrams, who must have been the one watching TV.

"The ambulance is needed on the parkway at the bridge for a two-car PIAA."

"10–4," I heard Nick say as I ran to the radio area. I nodded to him. "There are two EMTs responding. Tone out for an attendant and for a second crew to stand by until we know the number of injuries."

Nick and I must have been having similar thoughts. The bridge over the reservoir was under repair, and, in several places, the roadway was narrow and without adequate dividers.

"And put the chopper on standby," Nick added.

"10–4," Mark said, and began to tone out for additional personnel.

Nick and I quickly headed southbound on the parkway. It would take about three minutes to get to the accident scene despite the heavy holiday traffic.

The scanner in the rig shouted. "Car 305 to 639." Chuck Harding was calling police headquarters.

"Go ahead, 305."

"Get the chopper here fast, and we'll need at least two ambulances."

Nick and I glanced at each other. It was going to be a bad one, and he and I would be the first EMTs on the scene. The helicopter's flight nurses would be able to provide advanced life support when they arrived, but normally the helicopter had to warm up four or five minutes, then the flight time from the helipad at the trauma center was six to eight minutes.

"FPD to ambulance responding to the parkway."

"45–01 on."

"Be advised the officer at the scene reports serious injuries. The helicopter is in the air with an ETA of two minutes. Fire department's been dispatched for extrication."

"10–4," I said, then replaced the mike in the holder. "Holy shit," I said to Nick. "They must be in the air nearby. This must be our patients' lucky day."

As we approached the burning flares at the side of the road, the first thing we saw were four city police cars and vans that had pulled over to the side.

Nick glanced at me. "What the hell is going on here?" he said. "These cops must have been chasing someone. Maybe that's why the accident happened. The end of a high-speed chase."

"But we're forty miles from the city and their cars are facing toward it," I replied.

About fifty feet farther, in a small section without center divider, we could see the twisted wreckage of two cars that had obviously been involved in a high-speed head-on collision. Both cars were surrounded by men wearing black T-shirt uniforms with the legend URBAN SEARCH AND RESCUE TASK FORCE on the back.

"We have a fucking army," I said to Nick as we pulled

up to the scene. "I don't know what the hell they're doing here but I'm sure glad to see them."

One of the task force members came over to us as Nick and I got out of the rig. "You've got two patients," he reported. "There was no one else involved except the two drivers. My men have applied c-collars and have them both on oxygen. They'll assist you in any way you want. Four of our guys are EMTs." At my puzzled expression, he smiled and added, "We were on our way back from a training exercise at Camp Rogers when we saw the accident."

"God, am I glad you're here."

I headed toward one of the cars and Nick sprinted toward the other. As I approached the wreckage, I could see that the entire front of the car was collapsed in toward the driver. The windshield showed a spiderweb pattern with cracks radiating out from where the driver's head had obviously impacted on it. I approached the passenger side of the car where one of the task force members was crouched, assisting the patient. He quickly reported on the patient's condition, then got out of the car so that I could get in. Another black-shirted man was leaning in through the driver's side window, holding an oxygen mask over the face of an older woman who had been driving the vehicle. In the backseat, a young woman was holding head stabilization on the patient. She identified herself as Rita Lewis, a member of the Oakmont Ambulance Corps. "I thought I could help," she said, "but I'm not an EMT. When these guys arrived they told me to stay here, but maybe you'd better take over head stabilization."

"You're doing a fine job," I reassured her. "I'd appreciate it if you could hang in there until the helicopter team gets here so that I can stay in front with the patient."

"Okay," she responded. "I really want to help."

The driver was obviously in critical condition. Besides holding an oxygen mask, the task force member leaning in through the driver's side window was applying a large dressing in an attempt to stop the bleeding from a head laceration. Despite his efforts, blood was still streaming down the woman's face. Her bleeding nose was flattened and pushed to the side. Blood was seeping from her right eye, and both ocular areas were surrounded by blue-black discoloration—evidence that her eye sockets and possibly her skull had been fractured. The steering wheel was bent, suggesting severe chest trauma, and the dashboard was impacted against her knees. The woman was silent and, with the severity of her injuries, I didn't expect her to be conscious. I spoke to her anyway.

"My name is Ed," I said softly, trying not to cause any sudden movements. "I'm with Fairfax Ambulance and I'm going to help you. Can you tell me your name?"

"It's Kathleen Stephenson," she replied in a surprisingly strong voice. "Please get me out of here."

"We're waiting for the fire department to cut the car open," the black-shirted man said, still trying to staunch the bleeding from the woman's facial and head injuries. "We don't have sufficient access to get you out yet. And everyone calls me Press."

Amazed at our patient's level of consciousness, I said, "We're going to get you out as soon as we can." Will it be soon enough? I wondered. Meanwhile, there was little I could do for her. I took several trauma dressings from my crash kit, opened them, and assisted Press with bleeding control. All the while, Rita, Press, and I talked to Kathleen.

I had been with Kathleen for only about a minute

when I heard the pulsing throb of the helicopter as it landed on the parkway. Moments later Sharon Blackstone, one of the chopper's flight nurses, appeared.

I had known Sharon for more than twenty years. She had been an EMT with FVAC and had gone on to nursing school. Although Sharon was thoroughly competent, sometimes she seemed arrogant toward EMTs and cold toward patients. I had mixed feelings upon seeing her.

"Hi, Ed," she said warmly. "It's good to see you. We were just a few miles away on a training flight with some new navigation equipment when the call came in."

I marveled at the second fortunate coincidence for my patient. She and I were in luck. "Kathleen and I are very glad to see you."

I quickly gave Sharon a rundown of the situation and got out of the passenger seat so that she could get in and start an IV line. Replacing some of the fluid that Kathleen had lost was one of the few things that could be done for her.

I leaned into the back of the car. "Okay, Rita," I said. "I'll take over head stabilization if you'd like."

"Well," she said, "my arms *are* getting really sore and my back is killing me."

"I'm sorry," Kathleen said softly from the front. "Thanks." She's an amazing woman, I thought, worrying about Rita when she was obviously so badly hurt.

"Thanks a lot, Rita," I said, carefully taking her place behind Kathleen's head. "You did a good job and I really appreciate your help."

Relieved, Rita got out of the car and stretched her sore muscles. As I watched, Sharon quickly started an IV in Kathleen's arm, all the while talking and reassuring her.

"We're taking real good care of you," Sharon said. "Just try to relax as best you can and we'll have you out of here in a jiffy."

By now the firefighters had set up the jaws of life, also known as the Hurst Tool, and were ready to cut the car apart in order to get Kathleen out. Chief Bradley handed me a fire helmet and turnout coat and, with Sharon's help holding Kathleen's head, I struggled into the heavy, hot outfit. When I was ready, the chief ordered everyone else out of the car.

"Why?" Kathleen asked, her voice weaker.

"They're going to get you out of here, but there's going to be a lot of glass and sharp metal. They'll protect us really well, but anyone not needed will wait outside just to be safe."

"You?"

"I'm right here with you," I said.

They covered Kathleen and me with a tarp, then smashed the windshield. I reassured my patient continually as the shower of glass fragments bounced off the tarp covering us. As the firefighters prepared to cut the B post on the driver's side of the car with the giant pincers, Andy Johansen, one of the fire department officers, yelled to me, "Ed, don't move your left hand."

I glanced toward that hand. The cutter blades of the Hurst Tool were only a few millimeters from it as I stabilized Kathleen's head. Although I had been in the same position a number of times before during Hurst Tool extrications, I have never gotten over the terror of having a part of my body so close to those cutters as they chew through a steel post. Although I trust the firefighters completely, I can't help thinking that one slip and . . .

Continuing to hold head stabilization on my patient, I

turned my face away from the cutters, gritted my teeth, and closed my eyes. In a few seconds I heard the *pop* of the post as it was cut through. "Get me out of here," the woman said, over and over again. I knew that the fire-fighters were working as quickly as they could, but if prayers could help, I prayed.

After all of the posts were cut, the roof was removed, and I was finally able to straighten up. I'd been scrunched down in the backseat for about twenty minutes. The firefighters then used a hydraulic spreader to push the dashboard forward to free Kathleen's legs. During the time that it had taken to cut the car apart, Sharon had stood just outside of the passenger side, con-stantly talking to and comforting her patient, who had remained conscious throughout the long ordeal. As soon as she was allowed to, Sharon climbed back inside the vehicle to continue the only real treatment that any of us could offer—caring.

In a few more minutes Kathleen was free. She was quickly strapped to a long backboard and placed in the helicopter for her trip to the trauma center.

I hitched a ride back to headquarters in one of the police cars, picked up my computer, went home, and tried to work. Since I love my work, I usually find it an antidote to the bad feelings left over from such a difficult call. Much as I tried, however, I was finding it very hard to concentrate.

At about five thirty, my phone rang. "Ed," the unfa-miliar voice said, "this is Sharon. I just wanted to call and tell you that, despite all we could do, Kathleen died about half an hour ago, in the OR."

"Damn," I said. "It's so unfair that she had to be fully

conscious and aware of everything during that long, terrible extrication."

"Yeah. I agree. I just thought you'd want to know. There was nothing anyone could have done. The outcome was determined from the moment of the accident."

"Thanks so much for calling, Sharon. I really appreciate it. You were really great out there."

"So were you, Ed. I'm always happy to know it's you there at a scene. And she was a lucky woman to have someone like you talking to her and just caring."

"Thanks." I was amazed. This nurse whom I had considered cold had proven to be one of the most caring people I had dealt with. "How about the person in the other car? I never even found out whether he or she was transported."

"The driver of the other car was admitted in serious condition but he'll live. He has massive chest injuries and an open tib-fib but he never lost consciousness either. He says that he swerved to avoid hitting an animal and crossed into Kathleen's lane. She never had a chance."

"Yeah." I sighed.

"So, Ed, take it easy and get some counseling if you need it. That was a really bad one."

"I will. Have a quiet day," I said, repeating the standard phrase of emergency medical workers.

"You too." She hung up, leaving me feeling a deep sadness for Kathleen.

I had dealt with bad calls many times before and knew that my feelings would pass. I would talk about it with other EMTs; maybe even joke about it. Best of all, I would share my feelings with Joan, and that would be a tremendous help. I wondered, as I had often before, how full-time, inner-city EMTs are able to deal with the tremendous number of bad calls that they get. At least, I've often thought, as a volunteer in a suburban area, the really bad ones are relatively infrequent—maybe three or four a year.

Suddenly "Prescott Rescue to all home units. We have a report of a child struck by a car on Hickory Road at the top of the hill."

Ray Gilbert had rushed over to his friend C.J.'s house to show off the in-line skates that his mom and dad had given him for his birthday. Although his birthday wasn't until that Monday, his folks had seen no reason to keep him waiting, so they gave the skates to him early. "Hey, C.J., come with me while I try them out," he said.

"Okay, Ray. Just a minute while I grab my helmet and pads."

"Nah, we don't need them. I left mine at home. We'll just skate around the block a few times. There's no traffic."

"Okay," C.J. answered, grabbing his skates. He and Ray had been in-line skating for about a year, and neither of them had ever gotten hurt. They usually wore their protective gear only because their parents insisted on it.

They skated around the block a few times but quickly got bored. As they approached the intersection of Hemlock Way and Hickory Road, they saw a truck approach the intersection, lumbering up the hill. "Hey, Ray," C.J. yelled. "Let's grab onto the back of the truck and let it pull us up the hill."

"Great idea," Ray replied as the vehicle slowly rumbled through the intersection.

The two boys grabbed onto the back of the truck and

crouched so that the driver couldn't see them in his rearview mirror. As the truck crested the hill about halfway down Hickory, it began to pick up speed. "We'd better let go," C.J. yelled, becoming frightened. The two boys released their hold on the truck, and C.J. skated off onto the grass. Ray's left skate, however, struck a pothole. Momentarily off balance, the boy stumbled into the path of a car traveling in the opposite direction. He never felt the impact that crushed his chest and fractured his skull.

A child struck by a car. Since the accident was two blocks from my house, I dashed for my car without taking the time to call in. I roared down Hemlock and, as I turned the corner onto Hickory, I saw the child lying in the middle of the road. Prescott Police Officer Mike Gold was running over to him with an oxygen tank, and Dick Ramirez, whom I recognized as one of my former EMT students, was kneeling at the child's head, holding head stabilization. I screeched to a stop, grabbed my crash kit, and ran over to the child—a young boy wearing in-line skates, who was lying on his back staring up at the sky.

"What have you got, Dick?" I asked as Mike opened the valve on the oxygen tank and placed the mask over the boy's face. I saw that the boy had a massive laceration to the front of his scalp, which was bleeding freely. Mike opened a trauma dressing and pressed it gently against the wound.

"I don't know, Ed. I just got here. He doesn't seem to be responsive."

I checked the boy's mouth to be sure he had an adequate airway, then opened his shirt to check his breathing. I swallowed hard. The boy's entire chest, which was rising and falling deeply, was blue-black. The child was making a mewing sound with each breath. "What's your name, son?" I asked.

The boy silently stared up at the blue spring sky. I pinched the skin of his forearm, but he made no attempt to pull away. I pulled a blood pressure cuff out of my crash kit, wrapped it around his arm, and measured his blood pressure: 60 over 40. "This kid's in big trouble," I said to both men.

Prescott Police Officer Roy Zimmerman ran up. "The helicopter is on standby. What else do you need, Ed?"

"Get the chopper in the air," I replied.

Roy keyed his portable radio. "Car 703 to headquarters. Dispatch the helicopter."

"Ed," Dick said. "I don't like the way he's breathing."

I looked down at the boy. His breaths were too deep, ending with little sighs, and they were becoming irregular. "Roy, have you got a BVM in your car?"

"I'll get it."

Just as Roy ran back with the bag-valve mask, the boy took a deep breath, sighed, and stopped breathing. Roy handed me the mask. "You've got high-flow oxygen to the mask, Ed."

"Thanks, Roy."

I pulled the non-rebreather mask off the boy's face and replaced it with the BVM. Dick held the mask securely in place while I squeezed the bag. The boy's chest rose and fell. Dick's making a good seal with the mask, I thought idly. I'm glad I taught my students well. Working together, Dick and I continued to force the boy to breathe.

"Do you need an airway?" Dick asked. "I've got a set in my crash kit." He quickly told Roy where to find the equipment.

When Roy returned with Dick's kit, I selected an airway of the right size and tried to force the boy's mouth open so that I could insert the plastic device into his throat to keep his breathing passage open. His teeth were clenched so tightly together, however, that I couldn't force them apart. I looked at Dick. "It's no use," I said. "He probably has a brain injury that's causing his jaw to clench."

In a few minutes, paramedic Hugh Washington arrived.

"Hugh, we've got massive chest and head trauma. He's unresponsive to voice or pain and he's not breathing on his own," I reported.

"Take the mask off and I'll see if I can intubate him," Hugh said, preparing to place a breathing tube into the boy's throat.

I removed the mask and Hugh tried to open the boy's mouth. "I tried to insert an airway but he's clenching too hard," I said.

"I see. The flight nurses will have to put him down," Hugh said. Paramedics weren't allowed to use the drugs that flight nurses could use to paralyze the boy and get his mouth open. "Let's get him on the heart monitor and see what we've got. Let's just hope we don't have to do CPR."

I nodded as I looked at the boy's chest again. I suddenly felt sick and it was all I could do not to vomit. The idea of doing further violence to that small, thin, terribly injured chest was almost more than I could bear. I swallowed hard and continued doing the artificial ventilation that was needed to keep the boy alive.

Brenda Frost, a Prescott EMT who had arrived with Hugh, brought over the heart monitor, and Hugh attached the electrodes under the boy's collarbones and over his left lower ribs. The monitor showed a viable heart rhythm, and the boy had a carotid pulse. CPR would not be needed yet. Continuing to ventilate the boy with the BVM, we quickly immobilized him on a longboard and the ambulance transported him to the parking lot of nearby Alexander Hamilton Elementary School, where the helicopter was waiting to fly him to the trauma center. I knew that, if anyplace could save him, the trauma center could. I had little doubt, however, that he was going to die.

I had to walk home from the scene of the accident because my car was located in the middle of a police accident investigation scene and could not be moved. I called Joan and asked her to come over and pick me up. I told her about both of the calls, and she asked me several times during dinner that evening whether I was okay. "Sure," I replied. "The extrication was just an ordinary extrication and the kid was basically dead at the scene. You see one dead person, you've seen them all," I joked, shrugging off her concern. She looked at me doubtfully but didn't pursue the subject.

I was aware of no emotional reaction whatsoever that evening, but I was very tired and went to bed early. I felt completely exhausted and slept deeply until about 2:00 A.M., when I suddenly became wide awake. That was when the tapes began—the endless videotapes that you can't turn off. The endless replaying of the worst scenes of the day. Over and over I reexperienced the horror of possibly having to do CPR chest compressions on a young, already crushed chest; the dying woman's "Get me out of here, please" and the shock of seeing her crushed face.

The next day I found out that Ray had been declared dead at 12:40 that morning and that he would have been thirteen years old tomorrow. Although it was a warm, clear summer day, with the air filled with the smell of flowers and the songs of birds, it looked gray and dull to me. At times I found it difficult to carry on a conversation but at other times I felt perfectly normal. Mostly I felt an overwhelming fatigue and just wanted to sleep.

I'm writing this on the third day, with a tremendous sadness. There was a long article about Ray in our local paper. Suddenly he is not just a nameless body but a person, a twelve-year-old boy whom I tried to save but couldn't. To try to make some sense out of this, I'm writing about him and about Kathleen. Over the next few days, I will cry and I will recover from the shock of Saturday's double hit, and I will continue to do the incredibly rewarding unpaid job of a volunteer EMT.

The sense of hearing is one of the last senses lost when a person loses consciousness during a critical illness or after a bad accident. There are documented cases of people deeply anesthetized during surgery who had been able, after their recovery, to relate things that were said in the operating room. When I teach EMT classes, therefore, one of the things I emphasize is the importance of being careful about what you say when you are within a patient's range of hearing, even if he or she appears unconscious.

Until recently, however, I didn't really believe these stories. The idea of an unconscious person being able to hear just seemed a bit farfetched. In my gut I categorized these stories along with poltergeists and alien abductions, both of which are, according to some people, well documented.

At the monthly Prescott Rescue Squad business meetings, the recording secretary reads the letters received during the previous month. At a recent meeting the following letter was read:

To the members of the Prescott Rescue Squad who responded when I had my heart attack on the morning of April 5th.

I want to thank you all for your prompt, professional, and caring response to my wife's phone call to 911. I remember the terrible crushing pain in my chest and left arm, being unable to breathe, and the sudden weakness in my legs. I remember falling and everything going black. I don't know exactly when my heart stopped beating, but I remember someone pushing on my chest and someone holding a mask over my face, forcing me to breathe.

Although everything was black and I couldn't move or say anything, I heard everything that was being said. I am particularly grateful to the guy who was holding the mask over my face. He kept talking to me and telling me that I was going to make it. He was like a cheerleader. He kept saying "Come on, Gus, stay with us. Keep fighting." The others in the room called him Jack. I also remember feeling my whole body jerk when they shocked me. That must have been when my heart started beating again because they stopped doing CPR on me after that.

In the hospital, they gave me one of those clot-busting drugs and I was released after a week. My doctor tells me that, even though I was clinically dead,

*your actions brought me back to life and that there
was little permanent damage to my heart. He says that
I can expect to lead a normal life.*

*Again I want to thank Jack and the others on the
crew for saving my life and for the moral support that
they gave me even though I appeared to be dead.
Thanks to you I will be able to see my grandchildren
grow up. Prescott is very fortunate to have volunteers
like you to depend on in times of crisis.*

> *Sincerely yours,*
> *Gus Bernstein*

Even though I hadn't been on the crew for that save, I
left the meeting with tears in my eyes and a renewed
sense of awe at the power for doing good that I am fortunate to have as an EMT.

A sometimes frustrating aspect of being an EMT is
dealing with people who have waited much too long
before calling 911.

"How long have you been having these chest
pains, sir?"

"Oh, about three days."

"I see. And why did you call us today?"

"It's gotten a lot worse and I'm having trouble
breathing." Had this patient called sooner, his chances
for a quick and complete recovery would have been
much better.

But when medical emergencies occur in my own
family, often I am just as reluctant to call 911 as my
patients are.

A few months ago my ninety-one-year-old mother fell

as she and I were coming out of a restaurant. If I had been responding to a similar scene as an EMT, I would have thoroughly examined the patient, immobilized her, and transported her to the hospital. Even if she had wanted to refuse transport, I would have strongly urged her to allow us to take her to the hospital anyway.

But this was my mother. So after a cursory examination, I helped her get up and into my car, then drove her home. "If anything hurts tomorrow, I'll drive you to the emergency room," I said. Fortunately, she was not seriously injured.

Recently, however, I found out what it was like to call 911 myself.

For many years I have enjoyed international folk dancing, as has my sister, Esther. Recently, however, neither of us have danced very much. During the summer a very good folk dance group meets in Oakmont, in an old converted barn about half an hour away from my house. Deciding to go dancing one evening, I called Esther and asked if she would like to join me. Esther jumped at the invitation and, after meeting for a quick dinner, we drove to the barn in Oakmont.

Esther and I had a great time. We danced every dance, surprised that we still remembered the intricate steps after many years, giving no thought to the fact that we were a lot older and very much out of shape for some of the rigorous dances that we were doing.

About ten thirty, we began the troika—a Russian three-person dance. Esther was dancing between me and another man. We had just come to a particularly rigorous part of the dance when Esther suddenly sagged and became a dead weight between the two of us as we spun in a circle. I stopped turning and glanced at her, thinking that she had tripped. I quickly realized, however, that something was wrong. "I heard something snap," she said through her teeth as she clutched her right leg just above the ankle and sank to the floor.

As Esther writhed in pain, I examined her leg. There was no swelling or deformity and she was able to move her toes—a good sign. But I didn't have any idea of what to do. The other dancers gathered around, each offering his or her own suggestion.

"The same thing happened to me," one said. "You have to get up and walk it out."

That didn't sound like a good idea to me.

"It's her Achilles' tendon," another offered. "My brother-in-law had it. You'll need surgery."

"Why don't you drive her to the emergency room?" a third said.

One of the dancers came over with a towel containing ice cubes. "Here, put this ice on it," she ordered.

Yeah, cold, I thought. That's what I teach my EMT students. I took the ice and applied it to Esther's leg.

"Aren't you supposed to elevate it?" someone asked.

Yeah, right, elevate. I teach that also. "Yes," I said with all my EMT authority, "I was just about to do that. Does anyone have anything that we can put under her leg?"

People contributed various items, which I placed under Esther's leg to provide elevation. All right, what now? I thought. Apply cold, elevate, and . . . Suddenly it came to me. Transport was the next step. But I didn't have an ambulance with me. What to do?

"Why don't you call 911?" someone asked.

It had never occurred to me. And anyway, I had no idea what the emergency room would be able to do for her. Probably nothing, if it was only a muscle injury. But I had no idea of the extent of the injury, and Esther clearly could not walk. I would have to call 911. Leaving Esther in the care of other dancers, which I teach my students never to do since it can be considered patient abandonment, I went to the phone and dialed 911.

"911. What is your emergency?"

"I have an adult female with a possible torn Achilles' tendon or muscle injury in her right leg," I explained.

"Do you need an ambulance?"

"Yes," I replied. Did she think I was calling for her favorite recipe? I'm not a particularly tolerant man even under the best of circumstances, except when I'm with a patient, and this was my sister. She was hurt and needed help.

"What is your location?"

"The barn at the Oakmont Colony."

"What is the street address?" They obviously didn't have an advanced 911 system in which the address comes up on a screen.

I covered the mouthpiece of the phone. "Hey, someone, what's the address here?"

"There really isn't one," someone yelled back. "But everyone knows where it is."

I spoke into the phone's mouthpiece. "I'm told there is no street address. It's just called 'the barn' at the Oakmont Colony."

"We have to have a street address sir."

"I told you there is no street address," I hissed through gritted teeth. "Just tell the Oakmont Ambulance Corps to go to the barn. They'll know where it is."

"You'll have to calm down, sir. We can't help you if you get hysterical."

"I am calm," I shouted. "And I'm an EMT. Just send the damn ambulance."

"They have already been dispatched and they'll be there shortly."

"Thank you," I replied, slamming down the phone.

I rushed back to Esther. "They're on the way," I reported.

"Damn, it hurts," Esther said. "I hope the ambulance people know what to do."

"Well, they won't be able to do much except splint your leg and get you over to the hospital," I said. "If you're lucky, they'll be people that I've trained. A lot of the EMTs in this part of the county have had me for an instructor."

Within a few minutes, a familiar-looking young woman wearing a stethoscope around her neck and carrying a crash kit walked in. Spotting Esther with her leg elevated, she walked over to us. "Hi," she said, looking at me. "What are you doing here?"

The woman looked very familiar, but I couldn't remember where I knew her from. "This is my sister Esther. She hurt her leg while we were dancing. I'm sorry but I don't remember your name."

The woman looked at me incredulously, "I'm Carrie VanWyk," she said.

I stared at her in embarrassment. "I couldn't place you because you didn't step out of a helicopter in your uniform," I said, turning toward my sister. "Esther, you did better than getting one of my students. You got one of the best helicopter flight nurses in the county."

Over the six years since the helicopter service had been available to us, I had worked some really bad calls with Carrie. I even had ridden in the chopper to the hospital with her and my patient a few times. She was always calm, caring, and thoroughly professional, and it was always a pleasure to work with her.

"I didn't know that you were a volunteer," I said to Carrie.

"Yeah. I live in Oakmont and I've been a member of the Oakmont Ambulance Corps for years." Carrie turned to Esther. "The ambulance is on its way. I live close by so I came here directly. Now tell me what happened."

By the time the ambulance arrived, Carrie had gotten a complete history, had carefully examined Esther's leg, and had ascertained that my sister had no other injuries. When the ambulance arrived, Carrie and the rest of the crew quickly and competently splinted Esther's leg, moved her onto a stretcher, loaded her into the ambulance, and transported her to the closest hospital, St. Luke's Trauma Center. I followed the ambulance in my car, dimly remembering that I always tell people not to follow the rig when I'm transporting their friends or family but to meet us at the hospital.

At the hospital, I was asked to sign Esther in at the reception office while the ambulance crew wheeled her into the emergency room.

"What's the patient's name?" the receptionist asked me.

"Esther. Esther Herman," I replied.

"And her address?"

"Wait. No, it's Esther Ranz," I corrected.

The receptionist looked at me. "You're sure?" she asked sarcastically.

"Yeah. Herman was her maiden name."

"Her address?"

"Uh. It's in Hastings. At the top of the hill."

"You don't know her address?"

"Well, I know how to get there," I replied sheepishly.

"I think I'd better go in and get the information from the patient herself," the receptionist said, getting up. "Please wait here," she ordered as she left the room.

After waiting a few minutes, I went into the emergency room and found Esther being interviewed by the receptionist.

"Did you tell this lady that my name is Esther Ranz?" she asked me.

"Yeah," I responded, quizzically.

"It's Waters. Esther Waters, you turkey." She laughed.

"Oh, yeah."

I had forgotten that Esther had remarried three years ago.

I was happy to see several doctors and nurses I knew, and Esther was promptly cared for. The X rays showed a partial tear to the Achilles' tendon. Her lower leg was put into a cast and she was fitted for crutches. The recovery was prolonged and uncomfortable, and Esther can still tell when the weather is going to change. It was many months before we went dancing again.

Conclusion

When Joan became an EMT twelve years ago, para-medics, medical evacuation helicopters, and trauma centers were available in many areas of the United States but not yet in Fairfax. When I began my EMS career twenty-three years ago, these concepts were only in their infancy; only a relatively few years earlier, the local towing company had been responsible for removing victims from automobile wrecks, and the local funeral parlor transported them to the hospital in a hearse. If the patient died en route to the hospital, the hearse could easily change its destination.

When I joined the Fairfax Volunteer Ambulance Corps, we had a low-slung Cadillac ambulance that had originally been built as a hearse. There was not much room to move around in the vehicle, and it was virtually impossible to do CPR while transporting a patient. It was, however, the smoothest-riding vehicle that I have ever been in. It was wonderful for transporting patients with broken bones.

Soon we had to get rid of the Cadillac, however, in favor of large, truck- and van-type vehicles that met the new federal and state specifications for ambulances.

These new rigs had lots of space for carrying the increasing amount of equipment we were using and gave us much more room to work on our patients. Yet the patients could feel every crack in the pavement. Those ambulances were hell on patients with fractures.

Although back when I began all new FVAC members were required to become EMTs, our EMT training was not much more than advanced boy scout first aid. For a critically injured or sick patient, there was not much we could do except "scoop and run." Since there was no regional trauma center, we transported trauma patients to the local community hospital. The hospital then either called in a surgeon or attempted to stabilize the patient so that he or she could be transported by ambulance to a larger hospital that had appropriate specialists. In either case, the "golden hour" so critical for a patient's survival was frequently long gone by the time our patients received the treatment that they required for survival, and many died unnecessarily.

In those early days of EMS, for legal and other reasons, the medical profession was reluctant to allow any nonphysicians to use equipment or medical procedures that laypersons were not allowed to use. Doctors felt that it would amount to practicing medicine without a license. Even paramedics were always in direct communication with a medical control physician—a doctor willing to take responsibility for a medical procedure that was being performed without his or her immediate presence—and could do nothing on their own. The breakthrough for EMTs in Fairfax came when we were finally allowed to apply military antishock trousers (MAST) to trauma patients in shock, even though it was still only under the direct radio orders of a physician.

The next great advance was the introduction of portable, semiautomatic defibrillators for use by EMTs. Many studies had shown that, in cases of cardiac arrest, CPR is effective only when followed up by defibrillation—an electrical shock that "jump-starts" the heart. But special training and a medical control were needed, as well as funds to purchase the expensive machines. In Fairfax, a dedicated doctor started the program at a local hospital, and a large corporation that had a local facility that employed hundreds of workers contributed funds for defibrillators. Soon all Fairfax EMTs were trained as EMT-Ds and could use the defibrillators. I had my first defibrillation save only a few weeks after the program started.

Although a regional trauma center eventually was established, Fairfax EMTs still transported many serious trauma victims to the local community hospital because of the relatively long transport time to St. Luke's. Extricating victims from a serious automobile accident typically takes fifteen or twenty minutes, and we were reluctant to add an additional twenty- to thirty-minute ambulance transport time when the local community hospital was only five or ten minutes away.

The introduction of medical evacuation helicopters, run by the trauma center, was the next breakthrough in our ability to save lives. While an accident victim was being removed from a wrecked automobile, we could call for a helicopter. By the time we had the patient out of the vehicle, the chopper would be on the ground, able to transport the patient to the trauma center in less than ten minutes. Twenty-three years ago, it often took hours to get a patient into the operating room. Now the availability of the trauma center and helicopters allows us to get a trauma patient to the operating table in thirty minutes, only half of the "golden hour." And the helicopter flight nurses often begin advanced medical procedures at the scene, sometimes even before the patients are extricated.

For certain types of ambulance calls, EMTs alone can still do little more than "scoop and run." A person having a heart attack, for example, needs advanced medical intervention as soon as possible. Today paramedics can provide such medical treatment at the scene and during transport. For heart attacks, allergic reactions, and many other medical emergencies, paramedics can bring the emergency room to the patient. They can start intravenous lines, insert breathing tubes, and administer vitally needed medications.

It is difficult, if not impossible, to offer the level of care provided by paramedics on a volunteer basis, and, in an era of budget cutting, communities are reluctant to provide tax funds for emergency medical services that they have always obtained "free" from volunteers. At the present time, paid paramedics work together with volunteer EMTs in the Prescott Rescue Squad district. In Fairfax, an experimental program using volunteer paramedics working with volunteer EMTs is about to begin.

It is difficult to imagine future advances in on-the-scene trauma care that will equal those of the past twenty-three years. In the case of serious illnesses, however, I fully expect, before the end of my EMS career, to see all emergency medical responders capable of administering drugs within minutes of a heart attack or stroke, effectively bringing the trauma center to the patient and stopping those killers cold. In the meantime,

Joan and I will continue to respond and to do the best we can, even if it's only to hold a trembling hand or offer an encouraging word.

The Cast

Fairfax Volunteer Ambulance Corps
Radio Call GKL-642
County prefix 45

Emergency Medical Technicians
Nick Abrams—age thirty-four—works split shifts at the local Mobil station.

Stephanie DiMartino—age twenty-one—works in the local Kmart.

Bob Fiorella—age thirty-five—sells insurance and is able to respond to day calls when he's in the area.

Heather Franks—age twenty-four—works in the lunchroom of George Washington Elementary School and goes to college part time.

Tom Franks—age twenty-five—Heather's husband and a second-grade teacher at John Adams Elementary School in Fairfax.

Dave Hancock—age thirty-one—FVAC's Maintenance Officer—auto mechanic at a local auto-body shop.

Ed Herman—age fifty-nine—publisher and biotechnology specialist who works from his home. Radio call number 45–22.

Pam Kovacs—first lieutenant—age thirty-eight—works part time for a florist. Radio call number 45–12.

Joan Lloyd—age fifty-four—writer who works at home and responds to day calls. Radio call number 45–24.

Jack McCaffrey—age forty-five—professor at Fairfax Community College.

Sam Middleton—age twenty-seven—city firefighter—rides variable shifts as they fit into his schedule.

Steve Nesbitt—age fifty-one—drives a school bus for the Fairfax school system.

Phil Ortiz—age eighteen—became a first responder in the youth corps then, when he became eighteen, he advanced to the senior squad and became an EMT.

Linda Potemski—age thirty-nine—emergency room nurse at Fairfax Hospital and a longtime member of FVAC.

Fred Stevens—age forty-two—electrician with a local construction firm.

Marge Talbot—age thirty-four—CPA with a large accounting firm. Frequently works via computer modem and thus can occasionally respond to day calls.

Jill Tremonte—age twenty—dental assistant with the Fairfax Dental Group.

Pete Williamson—age twenty-five—professional paramedic with an EMS service in the city.

Probationary Members

Tim Babbett—age twenty-three—works for a local contractor—an EMT but hasn't yet become a full member of the corps.

Davida Herman—age nineteen—member of the youth group who graduated to the senior corps as a probationary member on her eighteenth birthday.

Dispatcher

Greg Horvath—age sixty-eight—retired plumber.

Fairfax Police Department

Radio Call ID GBY-639

Officers

Merve Berkowitz   car 317

Eileen Flynn   car 318

Chuck Harding   car 305

Will McAndrews   car 312

Stan Poritsky   car 308

Detective Irv Greenberg

Dispatcher

Mark Thomas

Fairfax Fire Department

Radio Call ID GCC-905

Members

Chief Paul Bradley

Lieutenant Patrick Connolly

Mike DeVito

Andy Johansen

Gerry McCarthy

Ken Stavitsky

Prescott Volunteer Fire Association Rescue Squad

Radio Call GVK-861

County prefix 21

Members

Paramedic Amy Chen
EMT Brenda Frost
EMT Ed Herman
EMT Jack Johnson
Driver Max Taylor
EMT Sally Walsh
Paramedic Hugh Washington

Prescott Police Department

Radio Call ID GRQ-325

Officers

Stan Garth   car 715
Mike Gold   car 706
Roy Zimmerman   car 703

At Fairfax General Hospital ER

Dr. Frank Margolis—emergency medicine specialist
Rosemary Harper, RN—emergency room head nurse
Patty Stewart, RN—emergency room nurse

At St. Luke's Trauma Center

Dr. Bruce Brown—third year resident in emergency medicine
Dr. Leonard Campbell—neonatalogist
Dr. Robert Englander—trauma specialist
Dr. Julie Gilmore—emergency room attending physician
Dr. Chris Holbein—psychiatrist

Dr. Maria Sanchez—pediatric resident
Dr. Janine Singh—emergency room attending physician

Carol Marks, RN—emergency room nurse and EMT
Erika Morely, RN—emergency room nurse
M.J. Kendall, RN—emergency room nurse
Steve Presley—X-ray technician

At St. Luke's Helicopter Service

Sharon Blackstone—flight nurse
Jeff Marks—helicopter pilot
Carrie VanWyk—flight nurse

Glossary

4 x 4s—Flat pieces of gauze measuring four inches by four inches, used to cover a wound beneath a bandage.

ALS (advanced life support)—The crew includes at least one paramedic who can perform the life support functions detailed below. See *paramedic*.

AOB—Alcohol on breath.

ASAP—As soon as possible.

backboard—A wooden board approximately six feet long and three feet wide. It is used both as a body splint to support the patient's body and as a lifting aid. Backboards are also called longboards or long spineboards.

BLS (basic life support)—Crew members can perform only the skills of an emergency medical technician with training in defibrillation (EMT-D), despite their level of training.

BP (blood pressure)—An indication of how strongly the heart is beating. Two numbers are usually given. (See *palp*.) The greater number, or systolic pressure, is the pressure when the heart muscle is contracting. The smaller number, or diastolic pressure, is the pressure when the heart muscle is relaxing. A

typical blood pressure might be stated as 120 over
80, meaning 120 systolic and 80 diastolic.

BVM (bag valve mask)—A device that forces air or pure
oxygen into a patient's lungs. It can be used during
CPR or to assist inadequate respirations.

call the code—In the hospital, the staff will continue to
work on a person even when the heart has stopped.
At some point, however, if the patient doesn't
revive, the decision is made to stop—to call the
code. Having made that difficult decision, the doctor
in charge will note the time of death.

CCU—Cardiac care unit.

cervical collar—A hard plastic, specially shaped bracing
device that surrounds a patient's neck to prevent
additional cervical (neck area) spinal damage. Also
called a c-collar.

closed fracture—One in which the skin is not broken.

contusion—Bruise.

COPD—Chronic obstructive pulmonary disease.

CPR (cardiopulmonary resuscitation)—The process of
using external means to circulate the blood, fill the
lungs with oxygen, or both.

crash kit—A container, often international orange, that
contains emergency supplies for an EMT to use
when assisting a patient. The crash kit, often called
a trauma kit, crash bag, or jump bag, contains such
supplies as dressings, bandages, scissors, lights,
equipment to take vital signs, and gloves. EMTs
often carry such a kit in their cars. One of the crash
kits carried in the ambulance is sometimes called a
megaduffel; it contains oxygen supplies, such as an
oxygen cylinder, BVM, oral and nasal airways, and

various types of masks, in addition to first-aid equipment.

defibrillator—A machine that can deliver an electrical shock to try to "jump-start" a heart that is in v-fib. (See below.) The defibrillator used by the Fairfax EMTs is semiautomatic. The machine assesses the rhythm and decides whether a shock is indicated. If so, it charges and requests that the EMT-D "press to shock." The manual defibrillator that the para-medics use merely shows rhythms on a screen and on a tape. From that information, the medics decide which combination of shock, medications, and/or CPR is indicated.

diaphoretic—Sweaty.

DOA—Dead on arrival.

EDP—Emotionally disturbed person.

EKG (electrocardiogram)—A tracing that indicates the electrical activity within the heart's muscle and nervous system.

EMS—Emergency medical services.

EMT—Emergency medical technician.

EMT-D—An EMT with added training in defibrillation. (See above.) All of the EMTs in FVAC are EMT-Ds.

ER—Emergency room.

ETA—Estimated time of arrival.

FGH—Fairfax General Hospital, the small community hospital that serves the fictional town of Fairfax. In addition to this hospital, down the parkway there is a county medical facility and trauma center.

FVAC—Abbreviation for the fictional Fairfax Volunteer Ambulance Corps. It is pronounced eff vac.

head blocks—Cubes of spongy material covered in heavy plastic that are placed on either side of a victim's head on a long backboard. Placed tightly against the ears and taped down, these blocks keep a patient from moving his or her head and prevent exacerbation of neck injury.

Heimlich maneuver—Choking maneuver popularized by Henry Heimlich and taught by the American Red Cross and the American Heart Association as part of their CPR courses. For a conscious person who can't talk, breathe, or speak, the "Heimlich Hug" can dislodge an object obstructing the airway.

hemothorax—A condition in which blood enters the chest cavity from an internal injury. This prevents a lung from expanding to draw in air.

hot off-load—When a helicopter is delivering a patient to the trauma center and has another call waiting, the pilot does not stop the engines. Rather, he leaves the blades turning while the first patient is off-loaded, so he can take off quickly and respond to the second call.

Hurst Tool—See *jaws of life* below.

hypovolemic shock—A potentially life-threatening condition (see *shock* below) resulting from severe blood or plasma loss.

intubation—Inserting a tube into a patient's trachea to maintain an open airway.

IV (intravenous line)—A tube inserted into a vein that allows a paramedic, nurse, or doctor to add fluid and/or medication directly into a patient's bloodstream.

jaws of life—A gasoline- or electrically powered hydraulic tool with several attachments that is used to pry metal from around an entrapped patient. The jaws, also known as the Hurst Tool, are usually used to disentangle a victim from a wrecked automobile.

KED (Kendrick Extrication Device)—A brand-name product. The KED is a plastic-covered, vertically slatted jacket used to immobilize the head, neck, and spine of an accident victim in order to minimize additional trauma while he or she is being moved.

Kling—A brand of roller gauze. Long strips of sterile gauze, prerolled and packaged, that are used to hold a dressing against a wound. Kling tends to adhere to itself, eliminating the need for ties or tape.

KVO—Keep vein open.

LOC—Either level of consciousness of loss of consciousness, depending on the situation.

logroll—To turn the body as a unit, to minimize the possibility of increasing any spinal injury. In order to transfer a patient lying on the ground to a backboard, we logroll him or her.

LZ (landing zone)—A helicopter needs a large open area, free of obstructions and overhead wires, in which to land to pick up a patient.

MAST (military antishock trousers)—Pants with inflatable bladders in each leg and the abdomen that can be pressurized like a BP cuff. Inflation is believed to slow the deterioration of a patient in shock. PASG (pneumatic antishock garment) is another acronym for the same apparatus. Currently the efficacy of this device is being debated.

MCI—Multiple casualty incident.

MVA—Motor vehicle accident.

neonatalogist—A doctor who specializes in newborns, especially those non–full-term babies with low birthweight.

normal sinus rhythm—The familiar lub-dub rhythm of

the heart. This is the normal rhythm of a functioning heart. (See *v-fib* below.)

occlusive dressing—An airtight covering used to keep air from entering a wound.

open fracture—One in which the skin is broken.

OR—Operating room.

oral airway—Technically called an oropharyngeal airway. This curved breathing tube is inserted into a patient's airway to hold the tongue away from the back of the throat and facilitate ventilations.

palp—Short for palpation. Obtaining a blood pressure by palp means that instead of using a stethoscope to listen to the patient's pulse at the inside of the elbow, the patient's radial pulse (see below) is felt while the BP cuff is deflated.

palpate—Touch a patient's body with light pressure.

paramedic—A member of the emergency medical services who can provide types of patient care beyond an EMT's training. Paramedic care may include invasive procedures such as starting IVs, administering medications, and intubating.

PCR (prehospital care report)—The report that our state requires us to fill out for every call.

PDAA—Property damage auto accident.

pediatric or pede bag—A crash bag containing supplies and equipment in smaller sizes to treat children and infants. In addition, the bag usually contains toys and distractions for younger patients.

PFA—Psychological first aid.

PIAA—Personal injury auto accident.

pneumothorax—A condition in which air enters the chest cavity, preventing a lung from expanding during normal breathing.

PO₂—An expression used to state the percentage of oxygen in the blood. This is a measure of how efficiently the lungs and circulatory system are working.

point-tenderness—Pain felt when an area of injury is touched or pressed.

prone—Lying facedown.

pronounce—The process of declaring a patient dead. In most states EMTs may not pronounce, whereas paramedics may.

pulses—Places in the body where an artery runs between a bone and the surface. Pulses can be felt with the fingertips. The radial pulse is found in the wrist, the carotid pulse in the neck, the femoral pulse in the groin, and pedal pulses in various locations in the feet.

Reeves—A stretcher consisting of a three-foot-wide assembly of six-foot-long plastic slats covered with plastic. A patient can be placed on the Reeves and the unit wrapped around the body. It keeps the spine supported while allowing the patient to be up-ended or carried at an angle through narrow hallways, over rough terrain, or down stairs. The Reeves has handles at each of the four corners and at the center of each long side, permitting a heavy patient to be lifted more easily.

RMA (refused medical attention)—A competent patient always has the right to refuse to let us care for him or her. It is, of course, our job, to try to convince an ill or injured person to let us help, but sometimes all our persuasion fails.

shock—The inability of the circulatory system to provide sufficient oxygenated blood to the vital organs.

SOB—Short of breath.

spider strap—An assembly of eight to ten connected straps used to secure a patient quickly to a longboard for transport.

stairchair—A narrow chair with small wheels on the two rear legs and handles for easy carrying. A conscious patient can be seated in the stairchair, belted in, and carried down a flight of stairs or wheeled across a smooth floor.

stat—Immediately. From the Latin *statim*.

Stokes basket—A heavy wire mesh basket large enough for a victim's entire body, often on a long backboard, to be placed for easier carrying over difficult terrain.

supine—Lying on the back, faceup.

tib-fib—A short form of tibia-fibula. The two bones of the lower leg. Since these bones are frequently broken at the same time, a break of the lower leg is referred to as a tib-fib fracture.

triage—The process of prioritizing patients when there are more patients than the medical personnel can care for. Assistance is given to those who can gain the most by care.

turnout gear—Coats, pants, hats, and boots made of heavy water- and fireproof material worn by firefighters. We in FVAC wear bright yellow, heavy, lined, weatherproof rain and snow jackets in bad weather.

v-fib—Short for ventricular fibrillation. During ventricular fibrillation, the heart's electrical impulses are disorganized and do not cause the heart to beat well enough to circulate blood throughout the body. Unless v-fib is converted to a normal rhythm, possibly by using a defibrillator, the patient will die.

vitals—Vital signs. Several measurable vitals indicate the stability of a sick or injured person. The vitals we measure are (1) BP (see above); (2) pulse rate and quality; (3) breathing rate and quality; (4) the appearance, temperature, and moistness of the skin; and (5) the response of the pupils of the eyes to light.

water gel—Heavy gauze impregnated with a water-based bacteriacide. These sterile bandages are placed on a burned area to both cool and protect the injury.

Additional Information

Ten-codes

Ten-codes are short code phrases used during radio transmissions that relay various pieces of information. These codes supposedly are easier to hear and understand over the radio than the actual words. They vary in meaning from department to department.

These codes are commonly used by both FVAC and Prescott Rescue:

10–1   Property damage auto accident.
10–2   Personal injury auto accident.
10–3   Illness.
10–4   I hear you and understand.
10–45 Obvious death. This is sometimes also abbreviated 10-100 or code 100.
10–99 (or code 99)   CPR in progress.

Additional code:

10–12 Police code that an officer uses to request backup.

The twenty-four-hour clock

In order to prevent confusion when reporting times, we do not use the terms A.M. and P.M. on our reports. Instead, we use a twenty-four-hour clock. Midnight is 00:00 and the times from one minute past midnight to noon are as they are on the regular clock. For example, 5:32 in the morning is 05:32.

From one minute past noon, 12:01, to one minute before midnight, the times are expressed as the clock time plus twelve. For example, 8:45 in the evening would be written as 20:45.

Authors' Note

We hope you enjoyed reading *Trauma Center* as much as we enjoyed writing it. We enjoy getting letters from people all over the country who share their stories, some of which have found their way into this book.

Since we are writing another book, we'd also be interested in learning the kind of stories you most enjoy so we can include those tales.

If you'd like to tell us your story or just let us know how you enjoyed the book, please write to us at:

> Ed Herman and Joan Lloyd
> PO Box 255
> Shrub Oak, NY 10588

or E-mail us at:

> JoanELloyd@AOL.com

LIGHTS AND SIREN

also by Joan E. Lloyd
& Edwin B. Herman

Dial 911 and they are there.

Emergency Medical Technicians are the first to arrive on the scene, and they are your lifeline to the ER. During those crucial first minutes, your life is in their hands. Here, in vivid detail from two EMT veterans, comes a firsthand account of the daily traumas, tragedies, and triumphs behind the lights and siren.

Published by Ivy Books.
Available in your local bookstore.

DIAL 911

also by Joan E. Lloyd & Edwin B. Herman

Imagine your worst fear.
A loved one falls to the floor, unconscious.
A car hurtles out of control.

You dial 911 and Emergency Medical Technicians answer the call. Now here are their incredible stories. DIAL 911 takes you inside the world of emergency medicine in a way you've never seen it before.

Published by Ivy Books.
Available in bookstores everywhere.

EMT
Beyond the Lights and Sirens

by Pat Foley

*Experience the rush of adrenaline
and the pain of loss.*

Pat Foley takes you inside the ambulance and on the road with volunteer rescue personnel. Witness the courage and compassion that makes the EMT an unsung hero in some of the most vital and compelling medical dramas of our time.

Published by Ivy Books.
Available in a bookstore near you.